THE KABBALAH BOOK OF SEX

For further information:

The Kabbalah Centre
155 E. 48th St., New York, NY 10017
1062 S. Robertson Blvd., Los Angeles, CA 90035

1.800.Kabbalah
www.kabbalah.com

First Edition
December 2006
Printed in USA
ISBN10: 1-57189-544-2
ISBN13: 978-1-57189-544-8

Design: HL Design (Hyun Min Lee) www.hldesignco.com

THE KABBALAH BOOK OF
SEX
& OTHER MYSTERIES OF THE UNIVERSE

YEHUDA BERG

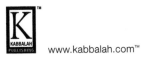

www.kabbalah.com™

ACKNOWLEDGMENTS

To the people who make my life better each and every day: my parents, the Rav and Karen; my brother Michael; my wife Michal and our children; and my dear friend Billy.

TABLE OF CONTENTS

BOOK ONE
IN SEARCH OF SEVENTH HEAVEN

WHAT'S IT ALL ABOUT?

It's all about sex. Everything. It always has been. From the creation of the universe to the mysteries of God, from the meaning of life to an actual formula for attaining never-ending fulfillment, understanding sex can help us understand it all.

In other words, when you know what sex is all about, you will know what life is all about. In turn, when you know what sex and life are all about, you will know how to ignite pleasure and infuse passion into your relationships, and we're talking about passion and pleasure that lasts a lifetime—with the same partner, no less!

Chances are you probably never knew sex was loaded with such majestic meaning and cosmic significance. According to the teachings of Kabbalah, it most definitely is.

The ancient wisdom of Kabbalah is about as straightforward as anything can possibly be on the subject of sex. And for good reason. Wise kabbalists throughout history tell us that a sexual act, far more intense and profound than you can possibly imagine, brought about the Big Bang creation of our universe about 15 billion years ago.

By the way, Kabbalah happens to be the oldest wisdom in the world. Abraham used it to grasp the interconnectedness of our universe (the oneness of God) some 4,000 years ago. Moses utilized Kabbalah to part the Red Sea and to achieve a temporary state of *heaven on Earth* during his ascension on Mount Sinai 3,400 years ago. Jesus was a kabbalist who tried to bring these powerful teachings to the masses more than 2,000 years ago. Plato borrowed from

Kabbalah. Later, Sir Isaac Newton, Henry More (Newton's teacher), and other great thinkers of the Renaissance drew from the ancient books of Kabbalah to begin the scientific revolution in the 17th and 18th centuries. In fact, one of Newton's greatest discoveries concerning the structure of white light is found in his personal copy of *The Zohar*, the most important book of Kabbalah. Newton's *Zohar*, which is still archived at Trinity College in Cambridge, was clearly an important source of inspiration.

Quite impressive.

In addition to possessing all the secrets of science and revealing all the mysteries of the natural world, Kabbalah also contains the secrets to great sex.

NO GUILT, NO SHAME

For far too long, religion has equated sex with shame, guilt, and embarrassment. Sex, from the standpoint of religion, has often been seen as a necessary evil that mankind was forced to endure in order to bear sons and daughters. Reay Tannahill, a scholar who wrote a book entitled *Sex in History*, says early Christian leaders equated sex with sin. She writes,

> *It was Augustine who epitomized a general feeling among the church fathers that the act of intercourse was fundamentally disgusting.*

The great Hebrew sage Maimonides taught that sexual intercourse was for procreation purposes *only*. Maimonides considered bodily pleasure a dreadful, vile thing.

Kabbalists held a different view. To the kabbalist, pleasing one's body was just as holy an action as pleasing one's soul. After all, it was the Creator who created *both* body and soul. Perhaps this is one reason why the religious establishment loathed and feared the kabbalists.

THE SACRED AND THE SEXUAL

Kabbalah promises us a fulfilling and wild sex life, which might be more than you dare to imagine. Because let's be honest: In most relationships, great sex lasts a year at most. Sex becomes routine. Sex becomes boring. For some, sex becomes no different than a household chore.

But sex was never meant to be that way. According to Kabbalah, God intended sex to be a never-ending, passionate experience, overflowing with profound pleasure and breathless excitement.

At this moment, you might be asking yourself,

God wants us to have hot, passionate sexual relationships?

You bet. Sex, according to Kabbalah, is the most powerful way to experience the Light of the Creator. It is also one of the most powerful ways to transform the world. That's right—sex can transform the world. The ancient kabbalists tell us that when the Earth moves beneath you during passionate lovemaking, spiritual worlds *also* tremble and move above you. So sex has a power that extends far beyond the door of the bedroom. Kabbalah reveals how our most intensely erotic moments reverberate throughout the Cosmos, just as a small stone tossed into still, deep water causes ripples that radiate outward.

We'll explore these ideas in greater detail later. For now, the critical question is this: If God intended for us to enjoy great sex, and if you just happen to agree with God, why doesn't great sex happen all the time in our relationships? Why has the sexual act been so deeply linked to guilt, shame, and abuse?

Enter *The Kabbalah Book of Sex*. The answer to this age-old question and the solution to the problem of passionless sex are what this book is all about.

TWO TALES OF DISCONNECTION

Meet Michael. Michael has just been to Seventh Heaven for the first time in his life. Seventh Heaven, as we'll soon find out, is a real place. It is a realm of pure, raw, naked energy. When you get there, when you touch Seventh Heaven, sex is wildly, madly magnificent.

It took Michael 41 years to get there. Michael reached Seventh Heaven courtesy of Kabbalah. Prior to his first trip, his pursuit of sexual pleasure was confined to chat rooms in cyberspace, his secretary's office, and the privacy of his bathroom. And, of course, it also included the occasional connection to his wife of 11 years, Meredith.

Michael tells it like it was:

> I was exactly like the character Kevin Spacey played in the movie *American Beauty*. After a few years of marriage, the electricity was gone. Sex became routine. For my wife, it was an obligation, like a mortgage payment due at the end of the month. I was having better sex with myself than I was having with her. I needed some excitement. So I flirted with my secretary, my wife's friends, and female clients—a lot of touching, kissing, and *explicit* sexual conversations. It was never my intention to cheat when I got married. But after a few years, I wasn't being sexually fulfilled at home.
>
> I was a selfish jerk, so I flirted whenever I could. My best friend at the time went all out. He cheated on his wife and slept with women all the time. Neither of us could find answers as to how

to keep sex as great as it was during the beginning of a relationship. Actually, let me correct that last statement. Looking back, it never even occurred to us to ask such questions. So we looked for cheap sexual excitement every chance we could.

Sexual boredom is a rampant problem in most monogamous relationships. Remaining faithful to one partner can often feel as if we are compromising, being forced to settle for less.

A COMPETITION

Meet Mark. At the time of the writing of this book, Mark is 45 years old. Mark's sex life began when he was 14. He was in ninth grade, attending school in the San Fernando Valley. During lunch break, he caught sight of a pretty girl wearing tight orange pants. Mark's friends told him her name was Robin and she was the *hottest* girl in the school. It didn't take long for Mark and Robin to become the class couple of the 9th grade and the class couple again in 12th grade. Their relationship lasted five years, until Mark read her diary. Robin had written that she'd had sex with a man named John, and then she'd had sex with one of John's friends immediately after. Mark freaked out when he read this. It didn't matter that Mark had had sex with more than 300 other women during his five years with Robin. He was overcome with jealousy and insecurity. He lost all trust in women at that point in his life. Sex was just a sport for him, instead of an opportunity for meaningful connection.

Mark recalls it:

> Sex was a race to the finish line. I competed with my friends to see who could get laid the most. I was having sex with two or three different girls every week. When I was a freshman in

college, I made a list. I had slept with 382 girls by that point. I even had a line item describing what happened with each girl: *Blow job in the library; two chicks going at it on the beach; two or three different girls in one day; two or three different girls at the same time.*

I was only 18. The real wildness hadn't even started yet. After college, I moved to New York and opened a modeling agency. It was the 1980s. I was making a lot of money. These girls were beyond good looking. Sex with a supermodel was incredible. Then something happened. The usual sex just wasn't getting me off anymore. So now it was two models at the same time. Even when my girlfriend was a Victoria's Secret model, I still had to have sex with her friends. When that wore off, it was sex with two chicks while doing lines of coke. Then it was sex on amyl nitrate. Then I had to jerk off while watching two girls do the same—all of us on crystal meth—in order to experience pleasure. Then, to get off, I had sex with two chicks while they had phone sex with strangers. After I ejaculated, I took more drugs and devised kinkier sex. Everything kept escalating, spiraling out of control. It wasn't the physical sensation of having two or three girls that excited me. It was the thought of it. Pushing the envelope was turning me on mentally.

The morning after these sexual romps, I would wake up in darkness. Depressed. Wiped out. I cannot even begin to tell you. I slept all my weekends away for a decade recuperating from those Friday nights.

Worse, I had absolutely no relationship with these women. Before I ejaculated, they were the most beautiful creatures God had ever created. But after my orgasm, they horrified me. I noticed hair on their arms. Or their nostrils were too big. Or their gums looked repulsive when they smiled—stupid little things that suddenly grossed me out and left me feeling disgusted. Nevertheless, the next night, after a line of coke and the promise of more perverted sex, they were again the most beautiful chicks in the world.

I remember finally getting really scared because everything was always escalating in order for me to get excited. I wondered, *How far would I really go? Would I soon allow someone—a man or woman—to put a strap on me, have sex with me, and then beat the shit out of me?*

Before it got that far, I actually wound up losing my business, losing everything. I was living in my car. I was nowhere. But it was a blessing. I found Kabbalah at that point in my life.

In the remainder of this book, you will find out why most, if not all of us, feel impelled to engage in kinkier forms of sex, escalating fantasies, and increasingly lewd thoughts to recapture feelings of sexual pleasure. But there is a way out. As you'll see, there is a way to understand how Kabbalah instilled a sense of magic in Michael and replaced routine and boredom with enchantment.

NO PAIN, NO GAIN

Great sex is going to require some hard work, discipline, and inner strength. First, you'll need to understand something about the origins of sex and the meaning of life if you genuinely want to bring about dramatic change. Second, knowing some of the fundamental principles of Kabbalah is a prerequisite to re-igniting the passions and pleasure that you felt when you first discovered sex. So this will take a bit of work, but the payoff is profound fulfillment of all your deepest desires. You might have to reread the chapters a few times, but this is a small price to pay for true transformation of your sex life.

The first half of this book lays down a solid foundation for understanding the origins of sex and its purpose. The second half provides you with practical tools to ignite your sex life. I personally recommend that you follow this order. We all like to jump ahead, but doing so will take the tools out of their proper context. Patience pays off, especially when it comes to sex.

A BIT ABOUT KABBALAH

Kabbalah is like a map of the universe's great mysteries. It's a collection of ancient insights and explanations that predates technology, biological science, quantum mechanics, and physics. Yet the greatest discoveries in those fields were already contained within it. Startling secrets of science and medicine were written down ages ago in its texts. For instance, Kabbalah explained the origins of heart disease 2,000 years before medical science arrived at the same conclusions in the 20th century. *The Zohar*, the major text of Kabbalah, said it quite clearly: Blockages caused by high levels of fat in our blood clog our arteries, and this causes both heart attacks and strokes. When a good friend of mine, a renowned cardiologist, read this passage of *The Zohar*, he said it literally blew his mind.

For many centuries, the secrets of Kabbalah were tightly guarded. Kabbalistic teachings were passed down in a secret tradition from teacher to student, from mentor to disciple. Kabbalah was restricted to a select, male-only minority for centuries. Only a privileged few managed to gain access to its ancient wisdom.

Some kabbalists believed that (along with the other powerful effects), Kabbalah study could unleash a sexual energy so potent, so powerful, that no unmarried man should be allowed access to it.

Happily for us, the veil has been lifted. In the year 1541, it was decreed by Moroccan Kabbalist Abraham Azulai, that Kabbalah could be studied by everyone and circulated everywhere. This great kabbalist actually said to spread Kabbalah in the open marketplace. From that point forward, kabbalists agreed that Kabbalah must be simplified and distributed so that even a six-year-old child could understand its teachings.

Would you believe many more centuries passed before Kabbalah finally reached the marketplace of ideas, which is why you are now able to read a simple and practical book on the subject of Sex and Kabbalah? Thankfully, all who want to explore its secrets are now invited. Today, lawyers, doctors, artists, salespeople, political leaders, homemakers, students, children, and millions of people from all faiths and backgrounds are eagerly discovering how they can use Kabbalah to bring Light into their lives.

Men and women of all ages, married and single, idealists and skeptics, can access the power switch. Personal background or beliefs have no bearing on the ability to apply these teachings to your life. Anyone with the passion for exploration can discover this ancient technology's capacity to enrich and elevate our modern existence.

But there is a caveat:

BE FOREWARNED:

Electricity brings great benefits to a city. All of our homes, hospitals, and businesses are dependent upon this great force. Just try to imagine city life powered by candlelight:

> No subways. No electric lights at home. No ovens. No refrig-erators. No home stereos. No blow dryers. No toasters. No TVs. No power in the hospitals. No street lights. No lights in downtown skyscrapers. No power to run the elevators. No Internet. No computers. No radio stations. No movie houses. No movies. Nothing but candles.

The advantages and comforts that electricity brings to us are almost indescribable. But it is also extremely dangerous to play with high-voltage wires. Electricity can cause great pain: Stick your finger in a wall socket, and you can kill yourself.

Likewise, Kabbalah's power must be respected. If your intent is to use this wisdom for selfish purposes, to indulge your own ego, this wisdom will prove to be useless. Doors will slam shut. You will short-circuit and wind up in the dark. Concepts will become confusing and utterly incomprehensible to you.

If, however, your goal is to enrich yourself and those around you spiritually, to remove chaos, pain, suffering, boredom, and empti-ness from life, then Kabbalah will light up your existence with an endless circuitry of power.

It's now time to begin our journey of discovery. Our destination: an exotic locale often referred to as Seventh Heaven.

A PLACE CALLED SEVENTH HEAVEN!

We live in a fantasy world, a world of illusion.
The great task in life is to find reality.
—Iris Murdoch

Seventh Heaven is a real place. It is not some remote fantasy in the minds of poets, philosophers, and incurable romantics. Seventh Heaven is an actual dimension built into the structure of the Cosmos, and it's older than time itself. This invisible realm is the source of our most intimate pleasures. Here passion is born, and sexual energy is summoned forth during wild lovemaking.

When you feel indescribable pleasure, you have made contact with this realm. When you reach a climax during lovemaking, the pleasure you experience flows from Seventh Heaven. When two people kiss and ecstasy engulfs them, the ecstasy is summoned forth from this dimension. It is the source of all the excitement, passion, and delight you experience during sex. The erogenous zones of your body, including your brain, are only antennae that tune into this realm and broadcast its pleasurable signal to your body.

It works like this: There is a curtain that divides reality into two realms, and these realms are known as:

- **The 1 Percent Illusion**

- **The 99 Percent Reality**

THE 1 PERCENT ILLUSION

This realm makes up only 1 percent of true reality. It is merely a shadow, a reflection of a vastly greater reality. You know this realm all too well. You laugh and cry in it. You sing and wail in it. You live and die in it. The 1 Percent Illusion is the world you experience with your five senses.

It is also the realm of boring, passionless sex.

THE 99 PERCENT REALITY

This realm, containing the rest of reality, is hidden. You cannot see or touch the 99 Percent Reality. Until now, you probably never had an inkling that it existed. Why is it so hard to detect? It lies on the other side of the curtain.

Yet every time you feel happiness, you somehow made contact with it. When inventors invent, when discoverers discover, they have connected to the 99 Percent. When poets write poems, when songwriters compose music, their works of art were already completed and waiting for them in the 99 Percent Reality. All the poet and songwriter did was make contact.

The same happens to you. Every time you connect with a principle presented in this book, your soul has successfully enjoined itself with the 99 Percent Reality—just as it is doing at this very moment! Every time you feel happiness, a sense of confidence, courage, or eroticism, your soul has accessed this hidden realm.

Put simply, all the happiness, pleasure, and wisdom we seek flows endlessly throughout the 99 Percent Reality.

Kabbalah has a word for all this happiness and wisdom.

That word is *Light*.

THE LIGHT DEFINED

The metaphor of *light* has been with us for centuries. It has meant different things in different contexts. For thousands of years, the idea of Light has been associated with any kind of breakthrough in human consciousness. The great religions refer to the *light of faith*. So do modern day preachers, who speak of seeing the light.

Even when characters on Saturday morning cartoons are struck by a great idea, what image appears over their heads? A light bulb, of course!

Kabbalah's definition of Light is the oldest, and the most specific in a profoundly simple way. Here it is: Whatever kind of wisdom you desire, whatever kind of happiness you may seek, whatever form of fulfillment you yearn for, they are *all* included in the kabbalistic concept of Light.

Light is an all-embracing word. It is all-inclusive. Just as sunlight contains all the colors of the rainbow, the Light that Kabbalah speaks of contains infinite varieties of joy, from the joy of chocolate—to the joy of great sex. If Michael and Meredith had had Light in their relationship, their sexual urges would have been fulfilled to the max! If Mark had Light in his life, he would never have needed a line of white powder to enhance his sex life. Sadness, self-loathing, and spiritless sex occur only when there is a lack of Light in one's life. It's as simple as that. Which leads us to consider . . .

WHERE THE LIGHT COMES FROM

This astounding Light radiates from a single, infinite Source that Kabbalah (and most other people) call God. In fact, Kabbalah tells us that all the religions of the world and all the spiritual doctrines of civilization are really referring to this awesome energy, this remarkable Light, when they speak of God.

Kabbalah does not speak directly of God for one good reason. God is a Force that is beyond infinite, beyond what the human mind can conceive. Put simply, a finite mind cannot possibly grasp an infinite Force.

Consider the sun. If you stood directly beside the nuclear furnace that is our sun, you'd burn up in a flash. Trying to grasp the concept of God is similar to trying to connect to the source of sunlight. On the other hand, the energy that flows from that nuclear furnace—sunlight—is a force you can embrace and connect with. In fact, sunlight is the very reason all of us exist. It gives us life. It gives us nourishment, power, and pleasure. Humanity receives the gift of physical life and nourishment from the light of the sun, not from the inner core and essence of this blazing fireball.

God works the same way, according to Kabbalah. The energy that flows from God is the Light that gives us life, joy, pleasure, inspiration, comfort, and sexual pleasure. This, in turn, leads us to ask . . .

WHERE IS THE LIGHT?

This awesome Light fills the Cosmos and permeates all reality. It saturates all human existence. It's within you. It's around you. In the same way that electricity permeates your home, Light permeates your life. In the same way that electricity keeps your heart beating and body functioning, Light gives existence to your body and soul. Disease, depression, and death occur when there is a deficiency of Light in your life.

All of which now leads us to the question that has plagued men and women throughout the ages, since the dawn of civilization, since the very first kiss and embrace in the night.

THE QUESTION:
If the Light is everywhere, why does the passion
and sexual energy in our relationships wane?

THE ANSWER:
Somehow, we disconnect from the Light.

DISCONNECTION CREATES SEXUAL DISCONTENTMENT

When you plug a lamp into a wall socket in your home, you access the force of electricity, and the light goes on. Unplug the lamp from its energy source, and darkness returns. Even when you are sitting in the dark, the electricity *is still there*. It never left.

Guess what? Life works precisely the same way.

The Light that enlivens our sex life turns off when we inadvertently disconnect ourselves from the 99 Percent Reality. When our connection to this unseen spiritual force of Light is severed, our sexual desires are unquenchable. We are unfulfilled. That's when people like Mark start escalating their sexual adventures. We start pushing the envelope. We begin looking elsewhere for sparks of Light. We are forced to find newer, edgier, riskier, wilder ways to experience pleasure to compensate for the yearning and darkness growing inside of us. Where do we often turn when we disconnect from the 99 Percent Realm in order to recapture pleasure?

Flirtation
Masturbation
Cyber sex
Phone sex
Pornography
Adultery
Three-way sex

Four-way sex
Chemically-enhanced sex

These are just some of the ways we try to fulfill our carnal cravings when traditional sex with the same partner just doesn't do it for us any longer.

There are also people who merely abstain from sex after the excitement has died. They compromise their desires, accepting a sexually unexciting way of life, thinking this is just another part of life's natural developments. So they try to find happiness in other areas of the relationship. Often they seek pleasure in business, careers, hobbies, or other endeavors.

But a kabbalist never settles for less. Never. According to Kabbalah, we can have it all! We were meant to have it all. That is the very purpose of Creation. Our job is to learn how to reconnect to that hidden realm known as the 99 Percent.

CONNECTION CREATES SEXUAL CONTENTMENT

When we connect to the 99 Percent Reality we experience happiness, including a whole lot of sexual enjoyment. When we're tapped in to this hidden reality, sexual excitement is powerful. Anticipation is breathless. Foreplay is electric. Orgasms knock your socks off.

The stronger your connection to this unseen source of power is, the more scintillating your sex life will become. Likewise, the weaker your connection is, the more boring and unexciting your sexual encounters will be.

Let's find out exactly how this works by peering behind the curtain that is concealing 99 percent of absolute reality.

A PEEK BEHIND
THE CURTAIN

If we could steal a glimpse behind the curtain and gaze into the 99 Percent Reality, here's what we would see: nine additional dimensions. When we include our physical universe, there are ten dimensions in total.

Let's stop here for a moment and think about this. Can you imagine telling someone 2,000 years ago that reality existed in ten dimensions? It would be like trying to explain a fax machine or the Internet to someone living in the 19th century. You'd be called a mystic or a madman, which is precisely what happened.

Two thousand years ago, when the kabbalists said reality existed in ten dimensions, the religious establishment called them crazy mystics and raving lunatics. But science has actually confirmed this ancient truth concerning ten dimensions. Far from being madmen, these kabbalists were extraordinary visionaries whose insights into the nature of reality, the creation of the universe, and even the cause of heart disease and strokes have been confirmed by modern-day physics and medical science.

Let's now explore the idea of hidden dimensions a bit further. Kabbalists gave us the following illustration to help us grasp the idea of a ten-dimensional reality.

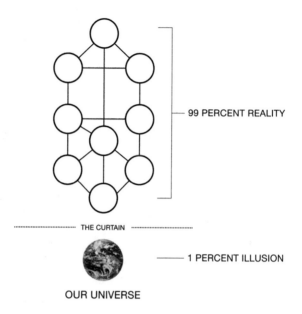

99 PERCENT REALITY

THE CURTAIN

1 PERCENT ILLUSION

OUR UNIVERSE

As you can see, the entire known universe, including the Earth, represents the 1 Percent Illusion. A *curtain* separates us from the other nine dimensions that make up the 99 Percent Reality. That curtain is formed by the limits of our five senses. Our five senses can detect only 1 percent of all reality.

But when we break through the curtain and enter these unseen dimensions, we connect to Light. You will learn how to do that soon enough. First, you must understand that just as a light bulb can shine in various degrees of brightness—25 watts, 100 watts, or 1,000 watts—the Light of the 99 Percent also has different intensities. The dimension known as Seventh Heaven provides the brightest Light of all when it comes to sexual relations.

LOCATING
SEVENTH HEAVEN

If you count seven dimensions upward, you will find the realm we access when sexual ecstasy flows into our lives. This is Seventh Heaven.

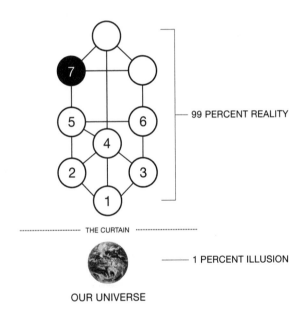

Kabbalists tell us that this realm is the storehouse, the repository, the fountainhead, the wellspring, the depot, the reservoir, the supply house, the treasure trove, and the stockpile of all the spiritual and sexual energy that permeates our entire existence. Each time we make contact with this dimension, we draw from this well of delight and experience sexual pleasure. We know it as an orgasm.

THE FULFILLMENT OF FOREPLAY

Before reaching orgasm, a human being experiences escalating pleasure, increasing excitement, and rapidly expanding thrills. This is called foreplay. During foreplay, your body and soul actually penetrate the curtain of this physical world and enter into the 99 Percent Reality. As your soul rises up through various dimensions, you experience rising pleasure. When your soul arrives at Seventh Heaven, your body goes wild. Orgasm is achieved as you taste a bit of the Divine. After your orgasm, your soul quickly descends back into this physical world. That's when you light up a cigarette, have a snack in the kitchen, cuddle, or roll over and fall asleep.

These hidden dimensions would have sounded an awful lot like mysticism a few thousand years ago. Remarkably, however, science continues to confirm what the ancient kabbalists revealed so many centuries ago.

SCIENCE
STUMBLES UPON
SEVENTH HEAVEN

Modern physicists focused on this ten-dimensional view of reality when they developed a remarkable new theory. The hypothesis supporting the existence of a Seventh Heaven is known as *superstring theory*, and it represents the cutting edge of scientific thought.

Let's keep this simple. Basically, *superstring theory* gives scientists a way to connect two great theories that each work in their respective field but otherwise do not relate to each other: *quantum mechanics* (which deals with the subatomic world of protons, electrons, and neutrons) and Einstein's general *theory of relativity* (which deals with the universe we perceive with our five senses).

Initially, *superstring theory's* claims of a ten-dimensional reality bewildered the scientific establishment. Renowned physicist John Schwarz of Caltech, one of the discoverers of this theory, explained in a PBS television documentary that the whole idea of ten dimensions was rather difficult to believe, even for his colleagues.

In the same program, physicist Amanda Peet stated,

> *People who've said that there were extra dimensions of space have been labeled as crackpots. Well, string theory really predicts it.*

Numerous experiments have now proved that validity of superstring theory and the idea of ten dimensions. Dr. Michio Kaku is an internationally recognized authority in theoretical physics. When he was introduced to Kabbalah's description of the ten dimensions and other kabbalistic concepts concerning the creation of the universe, he stated:

> I am a theoretical physicist. And I like to say that I walk in the footsteps of giants like Albert Einstein. Though I am not a philosopher, I am rather dazzled by the fact that many of the basic mysteries that we find in string theory seemed to be mirrored in Kabbalah.

Elaborating upon *string theory* further will not serve the subject matter of this book. However, what is intriguing and relevant concerning this whole idea of hidden dimensions is this: There is a reality we see and a reality we do not see. Kabbalah says the reality we see is merely an illusion, a shadow, and only 1 percent of all there is. The realm we do not see is true reality. Sex, according to Kabbalah, mirrors these two distinct realms.

Let's find out how.

DEFINING SEX

Humans are profoundly sexual beings. Kabbalah says our natural sexual urge is the engine that drives all human endeavors. Whether we recognize it or not, all of us have a tremendous innate energy, a deeply intense capacity for desire and physical pleasure. In fact, we are made of desire. We desire acceptance, love, fulfillment, excitement, wisdom, friendship, companionship, and recognition; we desire food, drink, pleasure, play, and great sex. According to kabbalists, the desire for sex is the strongest of all human desires.

Regardless of our religious upbringing, our personal philosophies, or our past experiences, all of us are, first and foremost, passionately sexual beings. But just as there are two realms—the 1 Percent Illusion and the 99 Percent Reality—there are also two kinds of sex:

- **1 Percent Sex**

- **99 Percent Sex**

1 PERCENT SEX

The "sex" that saturates advertising, magazines, and titillating television shows is passed off as *evocative of the real thing*.

It's nothing of the sort.

In fact, most of the sex we see around us in our culture isn't sex at all. It is just commerce in a tight black dress. Mass market, *sexy* imagery is to real sex what the squawk of a parrot is to the voice of Celine Dion or Andre Bocelli: a crude, inadequate imitation of the genuine article.

SEX AS SPORT

The kind of sexual Olympics our friend Mark competed in during high school is what we call *sex as sport*. It's all about the conquest. Nothing more. It's a notch in your belt, a trophy on your shelf. It's an "X" under the win column. There is no intent to develop and nurture a loving, sharing relationship.

This is sex in the most superficial, external sense of the word. This is 1 Percent Sex. It pleasures the body but leaves the heart and soul empty.

SEX AS A SELF-INDULGENT JOY RIDE

Carrie studied computer science and electronics in college and went on to become a computer networking engineer. Growing up, Carrie often wondered about life. She questioned the purpose of our existence, but never got any real answers.

Carrie shares her story:

> All my life I was looking for answers. I asked my parents, my teachers, "Why are we here?" There was no answer. I figured if life was really pointless, why not make the best of it and try to find happiness and joy? In my mind, it made perfect sense to have as much fun as possible. When I was 18, that's exactly what I wanted. Doing things that were forbidden really excited me. So as soon as I was outside the supervision of my parents, I went looking for the wildest times. I was open for it. I was ready for it. When you are open, it comes to you very easily.

> I met this girl who became my best friend, and she introduced me to guys at all these wild parties. I said to myself that I was now ready to try everything. I didn't care if it was drugs, sex with women, or orgies! One time, my girlfriend invited her boyfriend and me back to her apartment to party. We all took Ecstasy and got high. It was my first time. She started kissing me. The whole idea of a girl kissing me while her boyfriend watched made me fly to the sky. I would go outside myself and watch this whole scene. It turned me on because it was not allowed. My adrenaline went wild. We had oral sex, and then her boyfriend joined in. All I remember was wildness—arms, legs, lips—one big mishmash. It was like we were all one. It was amazing!

> Then I came down from the high and something came over me during the course of our three-way relationship. I started to become jealous of my best friend and her boyfriend. And she became jealous of me. And he became jealous of her. There were all these feelings of betrayal and mistrust and jealousy. I found myself bitchy and depressed all the time. I wanted so

much attention. Suddenly I wanted to hurt the person who I cared about the most. I was addicted to this relationship—the mental stimulation of the three-way sex, the touching, the excitement I was feeling for that moment, and the drugs, which multiplied everything by the thousands. Even though everything was getting more destructive and dark, I couldn't break the addiction! One day we came home from a party and my girlfriend fell asleep. Her boyfriend began touching me and we had sex while my best friend was asleep in the same bed. I knew it was wrong, that it was forbidden, but that was what turned me on. Our friendship was destroyed after that night. She couldn't handle it.

This three-way relationship provided us with great sex, but at the same time, it had turned into something very self-destructive! This story repeated itself over and over again in my life. The beginning of the relationship and the wild sex was amazing, but then it turned dark and destructive until my heart was broken. I couldn't trust anyone anymore. It got to the point where all the pain, damage, and hurt prevented me from getting high. No amount of drugs or sex could excite me any more.

I got a job as a computer engineer and had an important position. I dressed nicely during the day, and I was the one person in the company who was looked at with so much potential because I was so young and full of promise. That was during the day. At night, I was a slut. I had sex with anyone. I led a double life. The pain of this life eventually became so unbearable I stopped eating for half a year. I stayed at home depressed for six months. These crashes took me to very, very dark places.

Carrie is unusual not because of her sexual escapades, but rather because she connected the dots. What does this mean? Carrie had a sense that her crashes, her bouts of depression, and her feelings of revenge were somehow tied to her actions. Most people fail to connect the dots. We don't relate our dark moments to our own previous behavior. We see chaos instead of order. We believe life is random instead of purposeful. Carrie's insight—that her behavior was by some means contributing to her own pain—helped her open up to the idea of studying Kabbalah.

SEX AS ACCEPTANCE

Kate's been studying Kabbalah for close to ten years. She is happily married with four children. Prior to Kabbalah, sex did not signify true love for Kate. It was purely physical and shallow. There was no depth to the deed. As Kate puts it:

Sex was never about me. I didn't care about myself. I equated sex with getting love. Sex validated me as a person, so I had no restrictions, no boundaries. The sky was the limit. It didn't matter, because it was so empty. Yet, the more sex I had the emptier I felt inside, and the more shame I felt about myself. It was a sad cycle, really.

My low self-esteem caused me to give myself away for nothing in the hopes that someone would discover who I was and love me for it. Instead, the opposite would happen, and I would be left in degrading situations and end up feeling worse about myself. Each time I thought, *maybe this time . . .* but that time never came. It was so painful. And the worst part of it was that I did not even see what was happening; I did not see the pattern. I looked only at each situation separately. Ultimately, I believed I was not worth loving.

When I started to study Kabbalah, I started to really come to understand myself, the nature of the universe, and what sex was all about. I learned not to give myself up so freely. I found my dignity. I learned how to love myself and find joy and deep love and passion. What really surprised me was that before, a dozen different partners still left me feeling worthless and vacant. Now, I have total satisfaction with just one partner: my husband. If I had understood as a young girl what sex was truly about, I would have taken better care of myself until I found my present husband, who is truly my soul mate. I would have saved myself a lot of pain.

1 PERCENT SEX IS EMPTY SEX

The real adventure in sex is not in the number of partners, nor in the elaborately choreographed chase, no matter how stimulating and erotic that dance may be. According to Kabbalah, sex has the power to crackle electrically with intense energy and to provoke a heightened consciousness. But it's not enough to merely turn on. Animals are capable of physical arousal without any forethought. One must have the courage and focus to tune in as well.

Disconnected, tuned-out sex between self-absorbed partners is incomplete sex. It feels small. It shrinks physical intimacy to its most limited possibilities, rendering it hollow and quite often predictable, or even boring. Like a bad reproduction of an artistic masterpiece, it replicates but lacks the vision and inspiration that elevates the original to greatness.

Sex that's divorced from your inner self and from your partner prevents you from experiencing the kind of connections that evoke a sense of heaven here on Earth.

MOMENTARY SPARKS, THEN BLACKOUT!

Imagine you're alone in a dark room. Surrounding you are rows of lamps. Each time you turn on a lamp, it short-circuits. When a short circuit occurs, there is a momentary bright spark. But then the room is plunged back into darkness. The bulb's connection to the electrical current in the wall is short-lived because the bulb is defective. To ignite light in the room, you must run from one lamp to the next, turning each one on just to capture a bit of brightness.

Remember our friend Michael? Michael's flirting episodes were a lot like that. They were not true connections to the 99 Percent Reality; they were just momentary sparks in the dark. Carrie and Kate's episodes were equally short-lived in terms of generating fulfillment. Mark had the same problem. To recapture that moment of pleasure, Mark was forced to seek one short circuit after another, repeating the pattern endlessly, just to keep a little Light in his life. We all do this. It happens to us every day. The thrill wears off. Fun evaporates. The rush disappears. Pleasure gradually diminishes. When it happens, we rush off to find the next moment of immediate gratification instead of trying to learn how to make a lasting and permanent connection to the source of all pleasure: the 99 Percent.

If Mark knew how to make an ongoing connection to the Light, he would not have needed "three chicks" to excite him when "two chicks" no longer did it for him. Likewise, Mark would never have needed "two chicks" when his own girlfriend no longer aroused him. If Carrie had known how to connect to the 99 Percent, she would not have felt the urge to sleep with her girlfriend's boyfriend just to feel some pleasure.

Regarding these few last points . . .

GET THIS STRAIGHT RIGHT HERE, RIGHT NOW

Kabbalistically, we are not talking about morals or ethics when it comes to multiple partners in sex or any form of wild, kinky sex. In other words, Kabbalah is *not* saying that it is morally or ethically wrong to have two or three sexual partners at the same time. Make no mistake about it. Kabbalah does not deal in ethics. Kabbalah does not address morals. Kabbalah deals *only* with energy: specifically, how to connect to energy in the most powerful ways possible!

So the point is this: If Mark or Carrie had successfully connected themselves to the energy and Light of the 99 Percent Reality, they would have had no need for two or three partners to experience serious sexual excitement. A genuine connection to the 99 Percent would have delivered all the sexual pleasure Mark ever dreamed of with just his one partner. But, more important, the crashes and darkness that afflicted both Mark and Carrie afterward would have been avoided, for reasons we will discuss shortly.

You see, it's not about morals. It's about getting a better return on your investment. The only reason anyone tries alternative ways to experience increasing sexual pleasure, be it hardcore porn, an orgy, or sex on crystal meth, is that they are not as sexually fulfilled as they once were. And being fulfilled is why we were created in the first place. Kabbalah is merely a technology to show us *how* to achieve the most fulfillment possible *and keep it!*

After you've eaten a delicious meal that leaves you totally satiated, to the point where your stomach feels as if it were about to burst, do you really have a desire for two or three more meals at that precise moment? The only problem with 1 Percent Sex, according to Kabbalah, is that it leaves you feeling starving for more sexual excitement. There are also nasty side effects associated with 1 Percent Sex. It doesn't accomplish the original objective, which is constant fulfillment in one's life, and this is the reason kabbalists do not endorse it.

Having 1 Percent Sex confines you to this Earth. It lacks any form of deep soul connection. It's hot and passionate at the start, but it gets increasingly boring as time passes.

But there is a way to feel totally contented and fulfilled beyond measure.

99 PERCENT SEX

At the other end of the spectrum is 99 Percent Sex, or what we've come to call *great sex*. Great sex is messy, wild, and humming with multi-sensory delight. To paraphrase a popular sentiment, great sex is what many of us assume everyone else is having.

Great sex excites you to be bold, to be playful, and to shrug off your inhibitions. During great sex, you channel your primal impulses. You have moments when you may not even recognize your "regular self." Great sex feels like sex the first time, even after decades of being with the same person.

And 99 Percent Sex is totally transcendent. It takes you to Seventh Heaven and delivers joy and passion in endless amounts, pleasuring the body and fulfilling the soul.

You don't feel ashamed after engaging in 99 Percent Sex. You don't feel cold, dark, empty, weird, or indifferent to your partner after 99 Percent Sex. There is meaning, connection, and significance every step of the way, from the first kiss to the last embrace. There is the merging of two souls into one. And therein lies the key: the soul.

THE FIRST SECRET TO GREAT SEX

The key to great sex is making a connection to the 99 Percent Reality—specifically, to Seventh Heaven. How do we do that?

Our *soul* is one of the links that connects us to Seventh Heaven. Therefore, sex without soul can never deliver long-lasting pleasure and passion.

And how does one begin to have sex with soul? Sex with soul is 99 Percent Sex. Sex without soul is 1 Percent Sex, which takes into account the physical body and selfish immediate gratification. That's it. Sex with soul is 99 Percent Sex and takes into account someone far more important than your own self: *your partner!* Sex with soul also takes into consideration the rest of the universe and the meaning of life.

Let's examine these ideas further.

The experience of 99 Percent Sex begins with the understanding that there is an intimate connection between the vast universe out there and our personal sex life down here. This is a critically important idea in Kabbalah and thus worth repeating:

There is an intimate connection between the vast universe out there and our personal sex life down here.

What's the connection? You'll find that out in Book Two, which is coming up next. But first, let's review the key kabbalistic ideas presented in Book One.

THE KEY IDEAS OF BOOK ONE

- Of all human desires, the sexual urge is the strongest.

- The ultimate object of our desires is called *Light* (fulfillment, joy, and happiness, be it intellectual, social, sexual, emotional, spiritual or physical).

- The Light we seek from sex occupies a specific dimension in the 99 Percent Reality known as Seventh Heaven.

- When we connect to the 99 Percent Reality, we feel sexual delight and fulfillment.

- When we disconnect, we feel empty and frustrated. Somehow, we constantly short-circuit and sever our connection to this realm.

- There are two kinds of sex: 99 Percent Sex and 1 Percent Sex.

- Having 1 Percent Sex keeps you grounded in this physical world of pain and passionless sex. Experiencing 99 Percent Sex connects you to Seventh Heaven.

Those are the key points of our first section. All of which, if you stop and think about it . . .

INEVITABLY LEADS US TO THE FOLLOWING QUESTIONS:

How and why do we disconnect from Seventh Heaven?

How can we reestablish a lasting connection to this realm?

Why is there a Seventh Heaven in the first place?

Why does sex exist?

Why is it so hard to keep the Light on in our relationships?

Who designed the universe with ten dimensions, making it so difficult to connect ourselves to the 99 Percent?

Who created sex?

Who created the world?

Who created us?

And finally . . .

Why should we care?

BOOK TWO

IN THE BEGINNING ... THERE WAS SEX!

THE STORY OF CREATION

The underlying problem behind a lousy sex life and dysfunctional relationships, according to kabbalists, is that we do not know the answers to the following:

Who are we, really?
Where did we come from?
Why do men and women exist?
What is the meaning and purpose of our lives?
What is the role of sex in the physical and metaphysical scheme of things?
What tools are necessary to arouse true Light and sexual energy in our life?

As we find out the answers to these fundamental questions of existence, we can begin to experience truly great sex.

Contemplating the mysteries of the universe and the creation of the world may seem an odd topic of study in a book about sexual fulfillment. In Kabbalah, however, the cosmic and the erotic are intimately intertwined. That's right: Heaven and Earth are bound together in a single, stirring dance of creation. The world of two lovers locked in embrace mirrors the potential of the 1 Percent and 99 Percent to fuse into a single whole reality of endless delight and Light! When you see the connection, you will see the Light.

AS ABOVE, SO BELOW

The Zohar, the most important book of Kabbalah, says it all quite simply:

> *There is no stirring above until there is a stirring below.*

In other words, the Light that occupies the hidden dimensions of the 99 Percent Reality is awakened only through our actions down here in the 1 Percent Illusion. Our behavior determines whether or not Light flows into our realm to banish the darkness in our life. Our actions determine whether we are connected to the 99 Percent Reality or disconnected from it and stranded in the dark.

There are many behaviors that draw Light into our world. *Kindness. Sharing. Charity. Sacrifice. Overcoming one's ego. Prayer. Meditation. Sexual union.* These stirrings below cause a stirring of Light above. Sex just happens to be the most powerful way to access these unseen dimensions and bring Light into our world.

Here's the problem: There are sexual techniques that draw a tremendous amount of Light into our world. And there are techniques that cut us off from the source of all pleasure. What are those techniques? Why is sex the most powerful way to access or distance ourselves from the 99 Percent Reality?

The answer to these questions are found in a far away place, in a far away time . . . before the concept of time even existed.

Our answers await us at the very moment of Creation.

BEFORE THERE WAS AN ATOM OR AN ADAM

In exploring our universe's creation, the kabbalists found answers to fundamental questions about life, desire, intimacy, and sex. The forces and events that brought about the creation of the Cosmos have a direct impact upon our very own sex lives.

ORIGINS AND ORGASMS

Kabbalah says it clearly: A deep connection exists between the origins of the universe and the origins of an orgasm. Understanding the birth of the Cosmos will help us to understand what's really going on between the sheets.

We are now going to discover what Kabbalah has to say about the creation of the world. Not because we want to become wiser. Forget that. Nor is it because we want to develop a scientific understanding of the birth of the universe. The only reason we want to grasp how this world came into existence is that it will provide us with powerful knowledge to enrich our sex lives beyond even our own expectations.

So we begin this exploration of sex not with Michael flirting dangerously with his secretary in the middle of a work day, or Mark romping with a dozen supermodels in a hotel room, but in a "place" far more mysterious, and far more ancient.

We begin at the true beginning.

BEYOND THE CURTAIN

Long ago, Kabbalah opened the doorway to ultimate true reality. The kabbalists pulled back the curtain and peered beyond to behold the deepest, most hidden secrets of the universe.

Now take a deep breath before reading this next paragraph . . .

There is an ancient legend attributed to Kabbalah that told how four great sages once dared to peer beyond this curtain. Here's what happened to each of them:

1. The first sage died immediately because of the sights he saw.
2. The second sage went mad.
3. The third sage lost all faith in the existence of God after his experience.
4. Only the fourth sage who entered this forbidden dimension walked away safely, wiser, fulfilled, and with his body, soul, and mind intact.

In response to this legend, the religious establishment cautioned anyone who attempted to look behind the curtain. They warned the world never to enter into the wisdom of Kabbalah for fear of madness, heresy, or even death.

Well, it turns out this curtain had been left partly open for the last 2,000 years. This book draws that curtain wide. If you dare, you may now pass beyond the curtain and discover what only a few souls have ever known about the ultimate truth of our existence and the role that sex plays in the lives of men and women.

Will you go stark raving mad? Will you lose faith in God (if you had any to begin with), or die? Or will you walk away as you came, perhaps a bit more enlightened, wiser, and more sexually charged than you were before?

THE TRUTH BEHIND THE LEGEND

To conceal the real truth from the unworthy, the kabbalists always wrote in the poetic language of metaphor and riddles. The preceding legend is just that: a riddle! In other words, did a seeker truly lose his mind when he saw the truth? Did a sage really drop dead of hysteria caused by the visions he saw on the other side of the curtain? Most definitely they did not. In this legend, kabbalists are giving us a coded message: They are telling us something about ourselves.

What they are telling us is this:

Old habits are hard to lose. It is difficult for us to let go of preconceived notions. Narrow-minded beliefs are hard to surrender or change. It's easier to accept things as they are, no matter how much pain they cause us, than it is to fight to transform ourselves and change the world.

To grasp true reality, we must leave our own ideas, opinions, and belief systems at the door, just for the time being, so that we may be objective and unbiased when evaluating hidden knowledge about our origins.

We do not have to accept it as truth. In fact, we should always question everything and believe nothing. Belief is dangerous. It is unreliable. Results should be our only yardstick for determining what we know (not believe) to be true. As the great 18th century French philosopher Voltaire once stated,

> *Those who can make you believe absurdities can make you commit atrocities.*

For that very reason, kabbalists despise the concept of belief. They want you to *know*. And the only way to know is to test a principle. Apply it in the practical world. If it works, you won't have to believe. You will know.

So let's now unravel the riddle and discover the real lesson of the legend.

The four sages who utilized Kabbalah to peer beyond the curtain refer to the following truths:

1. If we hang onto our preconceived notions and resist growth, change, and spiritual wisdom, we'll wind up dying spiritually.
2. If we look at the world on a 1 Percent surface level only, the pointlessness, injustice, and chaos that we see will drive us to absolute madness.
3. If we judge the world solely by what we see, we will lose faith and never come to know the truth about God. We will not see the Divine design, purpose, and order that lies beneath the pain and chaos.
4. If we reach into the deepest levels of kabbalistic wisdom, we will discover answers and solutions to the world's problems (including an unfulfilling sex life), and we will embark on life feeling peaceful, sane, and fulfilled in body and soul.

Are you ready to take that first step? Okay . . . the curtain is now open. Let's go . . .

AND GOD SAID, "LET THERE BE LIGHT"

Before the first touch . . .
Before the first human whispers in the dark . . .
Before the first kiss in the night . . .
In the beginning, before anything existed, there was infinite
. . . *Energy!*

This Energy filled all reality. There was no Earth yet. No stars. No galaxies. There wasn't even a universe. Or a Big Bang.

There was only Energy. And this Energy was the only reality. There was nothing else. And it filled infinity, reaching as far as eternity.

Kabbalah calls this Energy . . . *the Light!*

WHY LIGHT?

The kabbalists chose the word *Light* for a very good reason. Like sunlight, which contains all the colors of the spectrum, Light was all-inclusive. It consisted of all the happiness, pleasure, joy, bliss, wisdom, and fulfillment the human mind can possibly conceive—and infinitely more than that, as well.

That's it. That's all there was: just an endless, infinite Light that embodied endless and infinite happiness.

Is it hard for you to imagine what infinite happiness feels like? Kabbalists told us 2,000 years ago that a single drop of this Light was actually 60 times more pleasurable than the greatest sexual orgasm you've ever had. Really. That's what they said. Now, if a single drop of Light was that powerful, imagine the power and pleasure of infinite Light! For eternity! Non-stop!

So that is the beginning. That is the starting point: infinite Light containing infinite pleasure.

THE NATURE OF THE LIGHT

This endless Light had one particular quality. This nature was to share all of its infinite happiness. In other words, the nature of good is to do good. The nature of sharing and happiness is to create and share happiness with someone else.

But here, in the realm of infinite Light, at the very beginning, that "someone" was missing. There was only Light. There was nothing else. So the Light decided to create someone to share with. After all, the concept of *sharing happiness* cannot become manifest without that act of making someone else happy. *Someone* has to receive the happiness in order for the sharing action to be expressed.

By the way, that is the first principle of Kabbalah you should master.

The Light of the Creator cannot manifest and express itself without a receiver.

So the Light decided to make someone happy.

That someone was *you!*

THE ONE AND ONLY CREATION

Yes, it was you. You were created by the Light to receive endless happiness. So was I. So was everybody else you know. So was everybody else you don't know. In fact, everyone who has ever breathed a molecule of air on this planet throughout history was created to receive endless happiness.

The Light created *all* the souls of humanity—past, present and future—in that one brief moment.

But guess what? All these souls were actually bound up into one great, unified soul. This is a bit abstract, but remember the metaphor of sunlight.

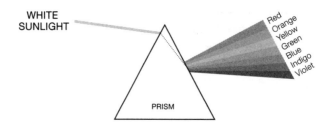

Sunlight includes all the colors of the rainbow. The colors are many, but they are also one.

Or consider a baseball team. There is only *one* team. But this one team is also made up of many players each playing different positions. Let's try one more example: Consider your body. You are one unique, individual person. But there are trillions upon trillions of single cells that work together to create the one and only you. Likewise, all the souls of humanity were like trillions of individual cells that made up the one giant unified Soul created by the Light. Each individual was unique but, *at the same time*, each individual helped to produce the *One Soul*.

THE ESSENCE OF THE SOUL

The One Soul had one singular characteristic. Only one. This unique trait is the key to understanding everything about life. So make sure you understand, as best as you can, what this one trait is.

The one trait is this:

DESIRE!

DESIRE IS ALL THERE IS

Because the Light was infinite, every kind of joy was contained within it. The only thing required to activate all this happiness was desire. When a desire is fulfilled, happiness is expressed in that moment of fulfillment.

If there is no desire, there is no happiness. Period. There's also not much of anything else. Men and women, adults and children, do not move a single finger unless there is first a desire to receive something.

> You work because you have a desire for cash, success, peace of mind, prosperity, or a new kitchen set.

> You eat because you have a desire to stay alive, or to experience the pleasure of eating something delicious.

> You compete in sports to fulfill a desire to experience the thrill of victory and achievement.

> You vacation to fulfill your desire for some serenity and a break from your routine.

> You enter into romantic relationships because of your desire to receive and give love.

> You watch TV and go to the movies to fulfill your desire to be entertained and experience enjoyment.

> You engage in sex to fulfill your desire for sexual pleasure.

So desire is the key to happiness.

To give expression to Itself, the Light created an infinite *Desire to Receive* all the joy the Light was radiating. This infinite *Desire to Receive* is the unified One Soul, of which everyone was and is a part.

LIGHT SHARES · · · · · · · · · · · THE SOUL RECEIVES

(+)   (-)

THE SIMPLICITY OF CREATION

The purpose behind all of Creation is actually simple. In fact, it is so simple that it can take a person a lifetime to grasp. We don't want to wait a lifetime. The Light's nature is an infinite ability to give pleasure. The Soul's nature is an infinite capacity to receive pleasure. Together, they form a synergy:

Creator and Creation
Cause and Effect
Emanation and Absorption
Sharer and Receiver
Provider of Good and Recipient of Good

This is what the original Creation was all about. Sharing happiness. Receiving happiness. And this is why you search for it 24/7. This is why human beings will stop at nothing to achieve happiness, however they may define it. Let's repeat this simple idea one more time:

A Force of Happiness created a Receiver in order to share and bestow endless happiness upon the Receiver. In other words, God created the Souls of Humanity to share Infinite Light with them.

So what happened? Why are we constantly looking for the happiness? What happened to it? You'll find that out in a moment. But first, do you sense something familiar about this relationship between the Light and the Soul?

IT SOUNDS A LOT LIKE SEX

In case you haven't noticed, there is a striking parallel between the Light-Soul relationship and the human sexual act.

The relationship between the Light and the One Soul was the ultimate sexual connection. For one thing, the pleasure that flowed between them was 60 times greater than the greatest sexual orgasm ever experienced by a human being. Not double the power. Not triple the intensity (which would probably kill the average human being). We are talking 60 TIMES MORE POWERFUL, INTENSE, AND PLEASURABLE!

And that is why the One Soul was created: To experience this Divine Pleasure for all eternity. Yes, the purpose of Creation is that simple. Life is that simple. We muddle up, and befuddle, over-intellectualize and over-complicate life in our pursuit of happiness. But if we stop for a moment and think about life, we realize we are all desires in motion seeking to fill ourselves with Light—be it in the form of wisdom, knowledge, money, friendship, love, or sexual ecstasy. Our problem is not the complexity of Creation and the purpose of life; it's our futile efforts at achieving the goal. We don't know how to consistently connect with the Light that was shining before this physical reality appeared. We're not happy. We're not sexually fulfilled. *What on Earth happened?*

Perhaps now is the perfect time to ask:

If the Light and the One Soul existed in perfect harmony and oneness, where, then, do we come into the picture?

How did our messy, imperfect, chaotic world burst forth from this flawless cosmic sexual synergy?

The answers to these questions lie in an extraordinary event that took place amid this oneness and bliss. A divorce!

Actually, think of it more like trial separation.

THE MISSING MAGIC KEY

In the first stage of Creation, the Light created one giant Soul in order to share endless pleasure with it.

In the next stage of Creation, the Light and the One Soul were suddenly separated, as distant from one another as east is from west. This spontaneous separation is why we find ourselves reading this book in a world of passionless sex. What caused the separation? There you have the most important question in the Cosmos! For the answer to this question is the ultimate, absolute, irrefutable key to understanding the mysteries of the universe.

Without this magic key, we couldn't possibly grasp the wisdom of Kabbalah or the meaning of our existence. Countless scholars throughout history have plumbed the depths of Kabbalah in search of its deepest secrets. Today there are stacks of books on the subject of Kabbalah in libraries and bookstores. Though they have uncovered poetic and mystical ideas, *none* have found this key.

Over the past 2,000 years, scientists, rabbis, priests, scholars and philosophers explored kabbalistic wisdom in the hopes of finding the secrets to life. All of them failed to find the magic key. All the books that were written on Kabbalah, all the meticulous research that has gone into the study of its sacred texts, all the scholarly papers authored on the subject, overlooked this carefully guarded key.

Until the end of the 19th century.

THE KABBALIST CALLED ASHLAG

He was born into this world in the year 1885. He left it in the year 1955. During his lifetime, he produced the most significant and historic commentaries on Kabbalah since the time of ancient Jerusalem. He was not merely a scholar. He was much more than a philosopher. He was not a sex therapist. He was a living kabbalist, one of the most prolific in all of history. His name was Yehuda Ashlag. This gifted kabbalist revealed the magic key so that, in our day, all of mankind could access this wisdom and apply it to life in a practical way. Where is this key?

It's in a minivan parked outside an apartment complex in midtown Manhattan.

LAWS OF ATTRACTION

I'm dating a woman now who, evidently, is unaware of it.
  —Garry Shandling

THE BLIND DATE

Liz lives in midtown Manhattan. She is a six-foot-tall, slender and vivacious 28 year old who loves travel and adventure. She seeks a man who is enterprising, wealthy, daring, and (she hopes) taller than she is. Liz loves Seinfeld reruns and Jaguar convertibles. She detests the idea of living in a suburban home with a manicured lawn, white picket fence, and a gaggle of kids tugging at her apron all day long. She adores the idea of taking off to Paris at a moment's notice. And she loves the hectic, fast-paced, high-rise, chrome-and-steel world that is Manhattan.

A colleague at work has arranged a blind date for Liz. Her date has just parked outside her apartment to pick her up.

Liz hears the knock at her door. She is filled with expectation. She opens the door and is quite startled. Actually, she is in shock. Standing in the doorway is a short, stocky, balding public accountant named Harvey. Before she can conjure up an excuse to cancel the evening, Harvey ushers her outside to his eight-passenger minivan. Liz knows she is past the point of no return, so she gets into the van. During their drive, short, stocky Harvey tells tall, leggy Liz all about himself.

Harvey wants a home in the Jersey suburbs and seven kids. He loves his steady nine-to-five job. Harvey likes to spend his weekends at home doing chores and some bookkeeping on the side for friends and family to make a few extra dollars. His favorite thing to watch on TV is reruns of Gilligan's Island. Harvey also has a fear of flying, so he has never been outside of the United States and doesn't plan to board an airplane for the rest of his living days.

Liz knows she's stuck for the evening, and she is dreading every minute of it. She is on the ultimate lousy date.

Although Liz and Harvey are sitting right beside each other in the van, they are actually worlds apart! Liz and Harvey are as far from one another as up is from down. This distance between them, however, has absolutely nothing to do with physical proximity. In other words, they might be close physically, but they are light years apart spiritually, in heart, mind, and soul.

The distance between them has to do with their opposite natures—their conflicting personal interests and desires—all the intangible qualities of their inner being.

Liz and Harvey have incompatible interests, contrasting desires, opposite goals and even dissimilar physical appearances.

Within this scenario, we find the long-sought-after *magic key* to understanding Kabbalah.

RAV ASHLAG
REVEALS THE KEY

As a blade slices and separates material things and divides them into two, so in the same way a "difference of form" or essence separates spiritual substances and divides them into two parts.
　—Rav Yehuda Ashlag

In spiritual realms, like attracts like! Sameness attracts sameness! The kabbalists, therefore, give us two key words along with their definitions.

closeness
1 : the quality or state of being similar
2 : the quality or state of being alike
3 : the quality or state of being the same (sameness)

distance
1 : dissimilar
2 : partly or totally unlike in nature, form, or quality
3 : not the same

In other words, the more two entities differ from one another, the further apart they are. The more similar they are to one another, the closer they are. This is called *the Law of Attraction*. The Law of Attraction is the magic key to understanding life and sex. When things are alike, they attract each other. They are close. When things are *not* alike, they repel, causing distance, creating separation.

You now have your magic key. Now let's apply this key to our original stage of Creation:

There is a Light that Shares.
There is a Soul that Receives.

In case you hadn't noticed, these are polar opposites. Sharing and Receiving are contrary to one another, as different as night and day. This complete state of dissimilarity suddenly caused a great separation between the Light and the One Soul. If you think about this, you'll see there is no way around it. The Light wants to Share. As a result, the Light created a Receiver in order to express the whole concept of sharing. But, in doing so, in creating an opposite form, the Light created an entity that was suddenly, vastly far away from Itself.

STAGE ONE

Light (+) Soul (-)

STAGE TWO

Light (+) · · · · · · · S E P A R A T I O N · · · · · · · Soul (-)

The Light and Soul possessed opposite forms, dissimilar qualities, incongruent characteristics, and diametrically opposing traits. For this reason, the Light and Soul were **divorced** from one another. Not because they couldn't get along, but because of natural law; the Law of Attraction that states: Like attracts like.

CASTAWAY

This situation seems pretty precarious. The Soul is suddenly cut off, alone, stranded. However, the great distance that now separates the Light from the Soul—*Fulfillment from Desire*—merely represents a work in progress.

The question now becomes: Can the Soul reconnect with the Light and regain closeness and unity with the Source of all fulfillment? After all, the Soul is a receiver by nature. Receiving is its essential quality.

This brings us to the end of Book Two.

THE KEY IDEAS OF BOOK TWO

Great sex is dependent upon us knowing how the world was created, the meaning of our existence, and the role that sex plays in our life.

Our actions in the 1 Percent Illusion determine the amount of Light that shines upon us from the 99 Percent Reality.

The origin of the universe is connected to the origin of the orgasm.

In the beginning there was only Light, which personifies and is the source of all happiness.

The Light created One infinite Soul to receive all the pleasure that the Light embodied. You were part of that original single Soul.

When the Light fulfilled the Soul, the joy was 60 times stronger than an orgasm. The relationship can best be described as Divine Sex.

The Law of Attraction is an irrevocable spiritual law that states like attracts like and dissimilar repels dissimilar.

The Light and Soul were separated because of their opposite natures: Sharing versus Receiving.

Before you turn the page and begin Book Three, you might be wondering,

> *Are the Light and Soul destined to remain apart because of their contrasting natures?*

Not a chance.

This situation is far from hopeless, for, as Dorothy eventually discovered during her perilous journey to the Land of Oz, the power to return home is already implanted within the Soul.

ADAM, EVE, AND THE DNA OF GOD

Parents of geniuses are great believers in heredity!
   —Unknown

If a child looks like his father, that's heredity; if he looks like the mailman, that's environment.
   —Unknown

DIVINE INHERITANCE

There is an old saying: The apple doesn't fall far from the tree. Science confirmed it with the discovery of the secrets of DNA and the genetic code. When the Light created the One Soul, the Soul inherited the genes of its Creator in the same way that children inherit physical and personality traits from their parents. Specifically, when the One Soul was created, its essential character was the *Desire to Receive*. However, the Soul also inherited a unique trait from the Light: namely the potential ability to Share.

The One Soul was conceived as a Receiver, but within its nature existed the possibility to Share and behave just like the Creator. Sounds simple enough. And it is that simple. Now here comes a tiny, little kabbalistic secret that will shake the traditional view of The Bible down to its very foundations.

THE SECRET:

The One Soul, whose essence is desire, is known by the code word *Eve*.

The sharing gene inherited by the Soul is known by the code word *Adam*.

The phrase *Adam and Eve* is really a code for the One Soul that possesses both a *Receiving* trait and an inherited, Godly, *Sharing* trait. Adam and Eve were not two physical people hanging out in some exotic earthly garden. Adam and Eve refer to the two character traits possessed by the One Soul: Receiving and the potential to Share and become like the Creator.

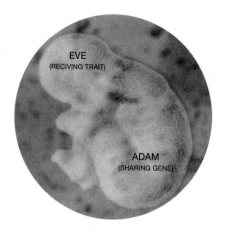

ONE SOUL

Here's some good news: According to the Law of Attraction, the Soul can reunite with the Light simply by emulating the Creator, simply by becoming similar in nature and behaving just like God. Remember, like attracts like. The question is: How?

HOW TO BECOME LIKE GOD

To unite with the Light, one must behave like the Light. To unite with God, one must become like God. So here is a key question, a question that holds the secret to becoming just like God:

QUESTION:

What does God never do?

ANSWER:

He never receives.

Therein is the problem. As long as the Soul continued to receive, its essence was opposite to that of the Creator, and thus it remained separated from the Light.

So the Soul attempted something radical.

THE SOUL STOPPED RECEIVING THE LIGHT!

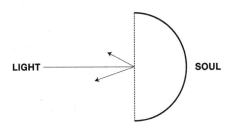

MISSION ACCOMPLISHED . . . *ALMOST!*

By stopping the Light and shutting down its receiving nature, the One Soul, also known as the Receiver, removed the one trait and one behavioral action that caused the separation: *receiving!* It was a smart play, a clever move. Except for one thing: When the Vessel stopped receiving the Light, it didn't remove *all* the Light. Why not, you ask? Consider a glass filled with milk. If you pour out all the liquid, a thin film of milky residue still remains in the glass. This is precisely what happened to the One Soul. When it stopped receiving, all the Light left, except for a tiny residue. **Because of this tiny residue, there was still a tiny *Desire to Receive* the Light within the Soul.**

CLOSE BUT NO CIGAR

Of course, the initial act of stopping the Light and shutting down the receiving nature made the Soul a heck of a lot more like the Light. In fact, 99 Percent of all Light left the Vessel. Indeed, 99 Percent of the Vessel's Receiving had now been eradicated. Naturally, this brought the Soul closer to the Light, but still not all the way home.

For that reason, there was still more action required by the Soul.

FINAL STEPS TO ETERNAL BLISS

The soul's step was twofold:

1) simply to resist the remaining 1 Percent residue of Light in order to achieve the ultimate objective of *completely* removing any kind of receiving from its nature, and

2) to share in order to develop the Sharing nature of the Creator.

Let's now examine the events that took place when the Soul first said stop!

RESISTANCE AND THE BIRTH OF A UNIVERSE

The Soul's action of stopping the Light is called *Resistance*. Why? The Soul is resisting the Light.

Naturally, the Light loved the Soul, loved it more than the human mind can ever comprehend. So the Light complied. The Light withdrew its infinite Energy when the Soul resisted the Light. The moment that Energy was withdrawn, an empty space suddenly emerged. The infinite Light had given birth to a finite point. This empty space was minuscule, just a single dot of darkness. And that is when something extraordinary happened: Suddenly, the Big Bang gave birth to our universe inside that microscopic empty point.

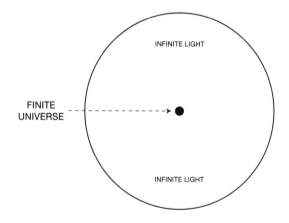

That detonation is science's Big Bang theory in the language of mysticism rather than physics. In other words, the moment the Light pulled back and created an empty, vacated point, *space* was created in the form of the Big Bang explosion that science says marks the birth of our universe. Remarkably, both science and Kabbalah offer identical accounts of the creation of the world.

A PLACE TO BECOME A CREATOR

This newly created finite space would now serve as an arena, a training ground where the Soul could learn, on its own, how to become like God. In simpler words, the Soul would now have its own unique place where it could resist the *remaining residue* of receiving that still remained and develop the nature of Sharing.

Remember, the first act of Resistance removed 99 Percent of the Light. This new playing field would give the Soul another opportunity to resist the left-over residue, the remaining 1 Percent of Receiving that still filled it.

Here's what happened.

TEN DRAWN DRAPES OF DARKNESS

To conceal its blazing Light, the Creator hung ten "curtains." Each successive curtain gradually reduced the brightness of the Light. The ten curtains were (and are) the Creator's way of diminishing the intensity of His Divine Light just enough for the world to occur.

Please follow this next idea carefully: Something amazing happened when ten curtains were put up. Each additional drape created an additional new dimension. Hence, ten curtains produced ten dimensions. The higher dimensions naturally contain more Light, as they are closer to the Source of all Light and are not concealed by as many curtains. The lowest dimension, obviously, contains the least Light and is our current home.

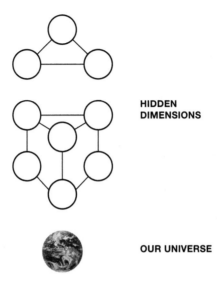

HIDDEN DIMENSIONS

OUR UNIVERSE

Welcome to our world of sex, drugs, and ancient scrolls.

THE STRUCTURE OF THE TEN DIMENSIONS

There is one more thing you need to know before we examine how human souls, love, and sex came into existence on Earth. You need to know how the Ten Dimensions are structured. They are grouped together as follows:

Three
Six
One

As we learned earlier, the magical place called Seventh Heaven is found in the upper realm of the Three Dimensions. Our physical world is the lone dimension at the very bottom. What then, are those middle six dimensions all about?

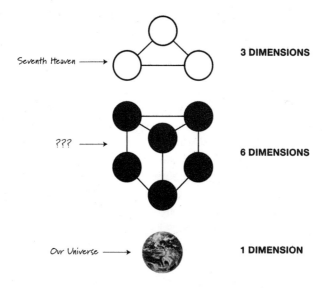

To find out, we must examine what is perhaps the most famous story in the history of human civilization: the story of Adam and Eve.

ADAM AND EVE

The Garden of Eden. The serpent. The apple. The fig leaf. The Fall. The biblical story of Adam and Eve is one of the most well known tales in the Judeo-Christian world. Concealed within the literal reading of Adam and Eve, a richly layered tapestry of meanings and spiritual and scientific truths has been revealed by the kabbalists for us to explore. Kabbalah delves deeply into metaphorical and spiritual territory, and its view of Adam and Eve in the Garden of Eden is anything but simple—and it has nothing at all to do with morality. It's a story, a code concealing wonderful truths about sex and life. It is also a scientific and spiritual blueprint of Creation.

Let's summarize the Garden of Eden story the way most of us first experienced it. The version of Creation that has made its way into our collective consciousness goes something like this:

> IN THE BEGINNING
> After creating the other living things of the Earth, God created Adam, the first man. But not wanting Adam to be alone, God made a partner, taken from Adam's rib. This was Eve, the first woman. God left the happy couple in the Garden of Eden with the instruction that while they could partake of all the delights they found there, including fruit from the Tree of Life, they were forbidden to eat from the Tree of Knowledge of Good and Evil, for the fruits were unripe and they would surely die.

> But someone else was in the Garden: the notorious serpent.

> Urged on by the seductive encouragement of the snake, Eve disobeyed. She plucked an apple from the forbidden tree and ate it. Then she offered the apple to Adam, enticing him to eat

it along with her. He did, and with that, their fleeting age of innocence was over.

Suddenly Adam and Eve realized they were naked, and they experienced their first shame. To cover up their bodies, Adam and Eve sewed fig leaves together and wore them.

God returned and saw what they had done. Angered by their disobedience, the Creator cursed them with mortality, a future of hard work and toiling on the land (Adam's labor), and with pain in childbirth (Eve's labor), before expelling them from the Garden.

Tearful and distraught, the couple descended from paradise.

There are variations, of course, but that's the story as many of us learned it. Let's now reveal some of the "problems" with this story.

TROUBLE IN PARADISE

If you haven't opened a Bible in some time, take a look at the book of Genesis and the story of Adam and Eve. You might be amazed to find that it's surprisingly brief, little more than five to ten pages in translation. Yet in every generation, it has engaged scholars, sparked imaginations, captivated artists, spawned heated arguments, divided the sexes, inspired endless interpretation, and been cited as the basis for a variety of religious and ideological crusades.

The protagonists of the story have frequently been used as political footballs. Eve is condemned as morally weak—a sinful seductress who brought about the fall of Man (Adam), placing blame for humankind's expulsion from Eden squarely on her shoulders.

This reading of Creation has inevitably attracted those seeking to limit women's rights and social power by linking all women to a biblical role stereotype that's sexually uncontrollable, disobedient, and cunning. This Eve becomes the burden and curse of an entire gender and, in the process, is a convenient scapegoat for Adam, who partook of the fruit she brought him.

This traditional take on the Adam and Eve story has led to women being:

mistreated and oppressed,
maligned and repressed,
controlled and possessed,
forcibly undressed,
pressured and stressed,

**empty and depressed, as well as
frustrated and distressed.**

DECONSTRUCTING GENESIS

From the point of view of the kabbalist (and for our purposes here), politicized interpretations and literal readings of the Creation story both seriously miss the mark. According to Kabbalah, the fable of Adam and Eve is just that—a fable—when taken at face value. But when we delve beneath the surface of the story, deeper truths begin to emerge.

THE ADAM AND EVE CODE

According to the kabbalists, the phrase *Adam and Eve* is code, a metaphor, which refers to a single, unified Soul that existed before our universe came into existence. As discussed in an earlier chapter, all the souls of humanity—including yours—were contained within this one entity. Imagine a spattering of tiny water droplets. Each individual bead of water embodies an individual soul, but if we gather all the drops together, they form a single pool of water.

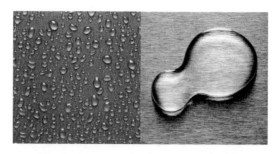

INDIVIDUAL BEADS OF WATER FORM ONE DROPLET

The Bible is not talking about two physical human beings made of flesh and blood. Rather, The Bible is referring to a non-physical Soul whose essential character consists of a huge Desire to Receive. What does this One Soul want to receive? It wants to receive all the endless joy that the Light is imparting. This gigantic desire is called Eve.

Within this Soul lies another potential trait, the DNA of God, which consists of a talent to behave like God. This trait is called Adam.

To summarize:

>   **Eve is the *Desire to Receive* in the One Soul.**
>
>   **Adam is the DNA and the potential to Share that exists in the One Soul.**

THE GARDEN OF EDEN CODE

Remember those six unidentified dimensions from a few pages back? Well, those six dimensions are actually the Garden of Eden.

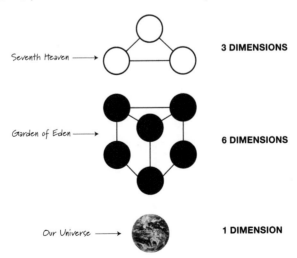

Seventh Heaven ⟶ **3 DIMENSIONS**

Garden of Eden ⟶ **6 DIMENSIONS**

Our Universe ⟶ **1 DIMENSION**

In biblical code, the Garden of Eden is where the One Soul hung out to resist the final residue of Light. This was the location and dimension where the Soul would attempt to complete the task of total resistance. The fact is that Eden was more like Madison Square Garden than a garden of paradise. Why? It was actually an arena where the greatest game in the history of the Cosmos would take place. Which leads us directly to the following questions (yes, questions play a big role in Kabbalah) . . .

If *Adam and Eve* is a term for the One Soul, and the Six Dimensions are the Garden of Eden, where do the apple and the serpent and the expulsion from paradise fit into the scheme of things? And perhaps the most provocative question of all:

Just what kind of game was played in the Garden of Eden?

This is where our story starts getting really dramatic and juicy. But first, let's summarize the key ideas presented in Book Three, for we have now reached the end of this section.

THE KEY IDEAS OF BOOK THREE

Although the Soul was created as a Receiver, it inherited the DNA of its Creator, which includes the potential to Share.

These two character traits of receiving and sharing are known by the code term Adam and Eve.

The Soul can reunite with the Light, according to the Law of Attraction, simply by behaving like the Light, which means sharing.

The Soul stopped receiving the Light so that it could have the opportunity to transform from being a Receiver into a Receiver that *Receives for the Sake of Sharing*. However, only 99 percent of the Light was resisted. The Soul had to resist the remaining residue.

The Light pulled back and created a tiny space, which includes our universe, giving the Soul a place to complete the final act of Resistance.

In the process of creating this tiny space, ten dimensions were formed.

The Garden of Eden and Seventh Heaven are both found within these hidden dimensions.

BOOK FOUR

SEX WITH A SERPENT AND THE FALL FROM PARADISE

THE GAME IN THE GARDEN

It's now time to erase the traditional story of Adam and Eve from our minds. It's a misunderstood metaphor that conceals ideas never before considered by the religious, scientific, or academic establishments. This is what actually took place:

The Soul is now in the Garden of Eden.

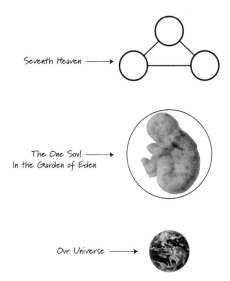

Seventh Heaven ⟶

The One Soul ⟶
In the Garden of Eden

Our Universe ⟶

In this game, the objective of the Soul is simply to nullify all receiving and resist the residue of Light. It all sounds simple enough, but then again, it's not. You see, something rather peculiar happened "up there" that led to you and me being down here, with you reading a book about how to enrich your sex life. To unravel this deep cosmic mystery, we must ask a critically important question:

> Why all these games? Why did the Soul have to undergo this whole process? If God has unlimited powers, why not create the One Soul in a perfected state of Godliness? Can't God do anything? Why not just create the Soul so that it is exactly like God from the get-go?

It's a valid question.

THE GREAT PRETENDER

Imagine getting a Ph.D. in psychology, but your father, a world-famous psychologist, did all your homework for you. He wrote your papers for you. He wrote your exams on your behalf. All you had to do was receive the diploma and doctorate on graduation day.

Are you really a psychologist? Are you really a practitioner of psychology in the truest sense? Or are you just a phony?

Let's now exchange the word *psychology* with *Godliness* in the above example:

> Imagine getting a Ph.D. in *Godliness*, but your Father, the true *God*, did all your homework for you, wrote all your exams, and all you had to do was receive the *Divinity* diploma and doctorate on graduation day.

Are you really God? Are you really a Creator in the true sense of the word? Most definitely, you are not. You are not genuinely similar to the Creator. You are a pretender. And pretending to resemble the Creator will never remove the space between the Soul and the Light. It has to be real. Genuine. Authentic.

THE POWER OF EARNING

Consequently, what the Soul desperately needed was the opportunity and experience of achieving that perfect state of being like God by virtue of its own effort. Only then could it genuinely know what it means to be similar to God in the true sense. Only then could the Soul attain a legitimate state of resembling its Creator.

This last statement is so profound, so lofty, you should take a few minutes to allow this epic notion to linger in your mind.

Now that your moment of pondering has passed, you should understand that there was only one way for the Soul to truly earn and be worthy of achieving a Godly state of being, a true state of NOT RECEIVING.

Enter the Serpent.

AN ANCIENT ADVERSARY

The Serpent is not really a slimy snake. The Serpent is another code word, a metaphor used to describe an opponent, an adversary: *a competing form of consciousness* that was created to combat and challenge the One Soul.

Struggling against the Serpent in an actual *game* gives the Soul something meaningful to resist. It's no different from building muscle. The harder a muscle resists an opposing force, the stronger it becomes. The Serpent would make *resisting* a difficult and therefore worthy challenge. This would, in turn, strengthen the God muscle within the Soul.

THE GAME

The actual game that the Adversary and Soul engaged in will be explained on two levels. The explanation of the first level of the game will be a simplified overview. Once you grasp that, we will uncover the details of the game on a deeper level.

Here's the game plan of both players:

> The objective of the Soul is to resist the remaining Light by resisting all Desire. Got that? Good.

> The objective of the Serpent is to tempt the Soul into receiving this Light and not resist it.

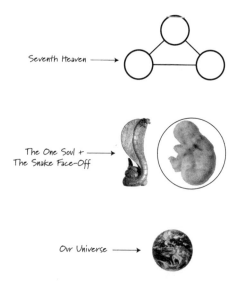

Seventh Heaven ——→

The One Soul + ——→
The Snake Face-Off

Our Universe ——→

IT'S ABOUT CONSCIOUSNESS

As we've now learned, the Garden of Eden was not a physical location. The Garden of Eden was a realm of pure and simple energy. Absolute consciousness. The same is true with the One Soul and the Serpent. They were not physical entities but rather entities of energy, beings of pure consciousness, which are far more real and authentic. Yes, it's hard to fathom a realm of pure consciousness while looking out on a world of frappucinos and SUVs, but the following explanation will simplify the key idea.

> The job of the Soul is to exercise free will. What is free will? Free will is the decision to receive or not receive. That's it. Nothing more.

> The Serpent represents the ultimate force of selfishness and receiving.

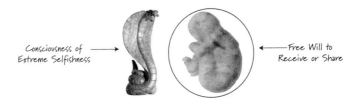

Consciousness of Extreme Selfishness →   ← Free Will to Receive or Share

So on a simple level the game is really a choice between receiving versus not receiving. On the surface, it's a slam-dunk decision. Obviously, the choice of not receiving will win the game for the Soul. Not so fast. It wasn't going to be that easy. The Serpent had a few tricks still to play. Let's now review the events that took place between the One Soul and the Serpent a long time ago, in a dimension far, far away . . .

THE CUNNING OF THE SERPENT

We're in the Garden of Eden. The Serpent is ready to do battle, but he has his work cut out for him. He will have to be cunning, calculating, and extremely deceptive.

The Serpent's task is a difficult one because, in the Garden of Eden, energy is the only reality. And this energy *vibrates* whenever truth is present. That's right, when truth is spoken, you can feel the vibrations in your very being. Lies and falsehoods are just as detectable. So it's relatively easy for the One Soul to distinguish between truth and deception, knowing that pulses of energy gleam throughout Eden when truth is spoken.

In response to this, the Serpent devises a clever plan. In a dimension where truth and trickery show their hand openly, the Serpent realizes that he must cover deception with a thin layer of truth to avoid detection. In other words, if a lie can be camouflaged with a coating of truth, it will dodge the "lie detector" that exists in Eden.

THE TRUTH ABOUT THE TREE

If you remember the literal story of Adam and Eve, God told the couple not to eat the unripe fruit from the *Tree of Knowledge of Good and Evil*, otherwise they would surely die. There was no physical apple tree in the Garden of Eden. The Tree refers to the Upper Three Dimensions. And the fruit is really Seventh Heaven.

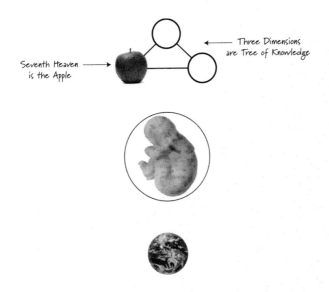

When God told Adam and Eve not to eat the unripe fruit of the tree, this meant the One Soul could not connect to this pleasure and receive it because that behavior is blatant Receiving. Receiving is the opposite nature of the Light. Receiving would cause even greater separation between the Light and Soul.

The Serpent knows this.

So here's what the clever rascal says:

THE SERPENT'S FIRST ARGUMENT

The Serpent tells the Soul that resisting the remaining residue of Light will take a lot of time and effort. There is a quicker, more efficient way in which the Soul can connect to the Light. The Serpent says the Soul CAN eat from the Tree and receive pleasure **providing** it does so with the pure awareness and intent that it receives pleasure for **the sole purpose of sharing** with the Creator. After all, nothing makes the Creator happier than seeing the Soul receive pleasure.

This is absolutely true.

And the vibration of this truth is made quite clear and evident to the One Soul.

Why is this true?

Follow this carefully, because it represents the heart and soul of Kabbalah and the ultimate purpose of life. The Serpent explains that when a person *Receives for the Sake of Sharing*, the act of receiving is **suddenly transformed into an action of sharing**. Let's take a look at an example.

A GIFT FOR DADDY

A little girl decides to make a new necktie for her Daddy. She draws a tie on a piece of paper. She colors it red, orange, brown, and purple and cuts it out. Naturally, she wants to share it with her father.

When her Daddy receives it, he makes a huge and wonderful fuss about it. His act of receiving **imparts** tremendous pleasure to his daughter.

This is called *Receiving for the Sake of Sharing*.

In other words, Dad has absolutely no desire or use for a paper tie whatsoever. He receives it because it will give tremendous joy to his daughter.

Something remarkable takes place:

> **The little girl shares by giving the paper tie to her father, and the father shares and gives pleasure to his child by <u>receiving</u> it.**

Both parties express the concept of sharing. They are identical in nature.

The Serpent uses this argument and spiritual truth to convince the Soul to connect directly to the Light.

THE SERPENT'S SECOND ARGUMENT

The Serpent explains to the Soul that if the Soul stops all forms of receiving, it will eventually become empty. After all, we learned earlier that Light could manifest only if there was a desire to receive it. If I want to share a bowl of steamed zucchini with you, but you absolutely despise green vegetables, can the concept of sharing take place? Not a chance. There has to be an actual desire for the object being shared.

The Serpent tells the Soul that without any form of Desire to Receive, the Light could never fill the Soul. Thus, instead of resisting the Desire to Receive, which would inevitably leave the Soul empty, the Serpent tells the Soul that Receiving for the Sake of Sharing would ensure a safe and eternal connection to the Light. The Soul would be receiving and sharing at the same time.

This is true.

The Serpent continues his argument by explaining the ultimate goal of the Soul. The explanation went something like this . . .

THE GOAL OF THE SOUL

The ultimate goal of the Soul is to learn how to Receive, not for itself but for the Sake of Sharing. By Receiving for the Sake of Sharing, the Soul automatically transforms the trait of Receiving into the trait of Sharing. Now the Light and the Soul *are both sharing*.

Guess what? According to the Law of Attraction, Light and Soul can now reunite because like attracts like. This is the key. This is the secret to achieving connection to the Light.

(Do not—*do not*—continue reading this chapter until this concept is firmly grasped in your mind. It holds the key to everything.)

The Serpent tells the One Soul that this is the ultimate way to connect to the Light.

This is true.

THE SERPENT'S THIRD ARGUMENT

In response to the warning that the Soul will "die" if it tastes the unripe fruit, the Serpent says this will happen only if the Soul receives the pleasure selfishly, for itself alone.

This is true.

After all, receiving is the opposite of the Light. Receiving would cause a separation and disconnection (death) between the Light and Soul. Therefore, the Serpent says, as long as the Soul connects to this realm for **sharing purposes only**, not only will the Soul not die, but paradise (the ultimate connection to the Light) will also become the Soul's possession for eternity.

This is true.

Now follow this next chain of events carefully:

CONNECTION!

The Soul realizes that everything the Serpent says is absolutely true. So the Soul decides to try it. Instead of resisting the remaining residue of Light, the Soul musters as much meditative power as possible and focuses on receiving this Light for the sake of sharing pleasure with the Creator. The Soul now connects to Seventh Heaven (otherwise known as Eve taking a bite of the apple).

Guess what? It works! The Soul achieves a connection to Seventh Heaven and experiences unimaginable pleasure. What's more, the Soul doesn't die. On the contrary, the Soul remains very much alive, in a state of bliss that is *60 times more powerful* than the greatest sexual orgasm. Apparently, the Serpent was right.

NOTHING SHAMEFUL, NOTHING SCANDALOUS

Kabbalists point out that the Soul's intention throughout this whole ordeal was honorable from the start. There was no act of disobedience, as stated in The Bible. There was nothing dishonorable about the Soul's behavior. That first "bite of the apple" was propelled by a pure impulse and the good intention to receive pleasure for the sake of sharing with the Creator.

Then again, we must also remember . . .

THE ROAD TO HELL IS PAVED WITH GOOD INTENTIONS

I'm just a soul whose intentions are good.
Oh lord, please don't let me be misunderstood.
    —The Animals

The kabbalists tell us that, in fact, the Serpent spoke only lies to the Soul. *Lies?* How could there be lies? The dazzling truth vibrations rippling throughout Eden when the Adversary spoke his words showed otherwise. The solution to this riddle is found in the biblical term "unripe fruit."

In the traditional biblical story God told Eve not to eat from the Tree of Knowledge—for its fruits were "unripe."

KABBALAH REVEALS A DEEP SECRET:

The term *unripe* **refers to the Soul**. It does not refer to a piece of fruit. In other words, the Soul consumed the awesome Light from Seventh Heaven **before** the Soul was ripe enough to handle the full impact. What do we mean by ripe? Specifically, we mean before the Soul's *Desire to Receive* was 100 percent expunged from its nature. Remember, instead of resisting the residue of Light and shutting down all desire, the Soul did the opposite. It received. Because of this, the connection was made prematurely, as you will see in the following example.

THE COKE ADDICT

A person who vows to refrain from a specific lust before he actually tastes of it will find it much easier to do so than a person who has already experienced the pleasure. For instance, if a person has never snorted cocaine, he'll find it easier to resist a line of coke than someone who has already gotten high from it. The second person requires far greater willpower to resist the temptation, because the white powder has already been in his system. This second person has already experienced the pleasure.

And so, the Kabbalist Rav Ashlag stated,

> The first person can obviously abstain himself from his lust once and forever. Which is not the case for the second person, who needs extra effort in order to withdraw gradually from his craving until he is completely free of it.

And, as you are about to see, the Serpent was keenly aware of this!

THE SECOND BITE

The Soul had never tasted of the "fruit" of Seventh Heaven when it first connected to it. Therefore, it was easy to take the first bite with the pure intention of imparting pleasure to the Creator. But something wild and unanticipated happened **after** the first bite. The pleasure of the first bite sent the Soul's remaining receiving nature careening wildly out of control. Remember, the Serpent told the Soul not to waste time Resisting the residue of Light. Instead of Resisting, the Serpent told the Soul to Receive but do so for the Sake of Sharing.

But do you know what happened? The Soul was suddenly compelled by an uncontrolled craving for more Light, more pleasure, once it had tasted the Light. It was like the seedlings of addiction. A Pandora's box was opened upon taking that first bite. Consequently, on the second bite, the Soul could not resist its *Desire to Receive*, for it had multiplied enormously.

THE SECOND BITE

The problem of the Second Bite can be understood on a more practical level. Consider sex. Before engaging in sexual intercourse, a man will often make a conscious decision to hold off as long as possible before reaching orgasm. The man's intention is pure. He is making an earnest attempt at postponing his own pleasure so that he can share more pleasure with his partner. When he has made the decision to hold off, he does not taste any pleasure at that time. However, as pleasure starts to engulf him during the initial stages of intercourse, the excitement becomes overwhelming. Suddenly, he abandons all his good intentions and comes to orgasm immediately.

This is exactly what happened to the Soul.

Rav Ashlag states:

> When the woman (referring to the Receiving aspect of the Soul) had not yet tasted the fruit, and she was totally in a state of Sharing, it was easy for her to eat the first bite with the pure intention of sharing pleasure with the Almighty.

> But after she had tasted it, she became bound by a strong craving for the fruit. She was no longer able to resist this craving. It was already out of her control. This is the meaning of the statement of our sages of blessed memory when they stated "they did eat unripe fruit."

As a result, during the Second Bite, the Soul could not *Receive for the Sake of Sharing*. Self-interest was awakened by tasting the initial unimaginable delight of Seventh Heaven. In other words, the Soul inhaled before it had acquired the full measure of strength to permanently rule over its receiving impulses. The *Desire to Receive* was not yet fully purged from its nature. The Soul connected prematurely to the pleasure of Seventh Heaven and thus the *Desire to Receive* skyrocketed during the Second Bite.

More Resistance was needed to eradicate the trait of Receiving. The First Bite was pure. The Second Bite was not.

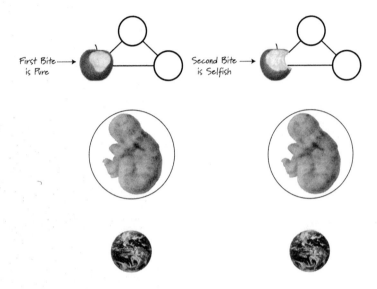

The crafty Serpent knew this from the very start. This is why the kabbalists say the Serpent spoke only lies.

THE ACTUAL GAME

Are you ready to go a bit deeper? Are you ready to flex your mental muscles in order to understand more about the shenanigans that took place in Eden? Let's do it.

The Serpent was brought into existence by the Creator to challenge us. The Serpent was not a hideous demonic creature. It was not the slithering snake that we learned about in Sunday school. The Serpent was actually an angel, a spiritual force and heavenly being made up of Divine Light, just as the One Soul was. It was a beautiful, compelling, angelic force.

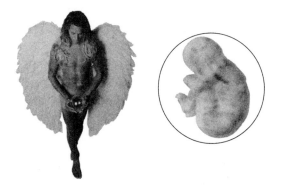

THE ADVERSARY + THE ONE SOUL FACE-OFF

And the game that was played between the Angel and the One Soul was the game called sex! Specifically, the connection that took place between the Soul and Seventh Heaven was really a sexual connection between the Adversary and the Soul, although it did not involve material bodies. It was sex on a spiritual level, in the realm of consciousness. But make no mistake: It was sex nonetheless.

BIGGER DESIRE AND THE BIRTH OF SELFISHNESS

When the Soul partook of the Second Bite, that Soul's desire skyrocketed because of the unimaginable pleasure it had experienced. This is like a person who is dieting. The dieter keeps to the diet all day long. Evening rolls around, and suddenly cravings for something sweet start intensifying. If the dieter cheats and takes a tiny bite of chocolate, the pleasure often overcomes the person and he or she winds up gorging on chocolate. If, however, that first bite of chocolate is avoided, the dieter usually has the willpower to resist cheating for the rest of the evening.

It's that initial small taste that leads to a massive meltdown. It causes our desire to skyrocket. Not only do we eat the tiny, delicious, decadent piece of chocolate, we must also consume a pound of Oreo cookies in order to appease our out-of-control craving.

The same thing happened to the Soul. When it tasted the first bite, its desire skyrocketed. The Soul was then forced to eat the equivalent of a pound of Oreo cookies in the form of Light during that Second Bite. Wow. Suddenly a massive surge of energy was ingested by the Soul.

In other words, during the spiritual sexual encounter between the Soul and the Adversary, the Soul was initially receiving pleasure for the sole purpose of Sharing. However, as the Soul experienced this sexual pleasure, it suddenly shifted its consciousness from Sharing into selfish desire. Now it was Receiving for Itself Alone. Now it was out of control. This would have shattering consequences.

ORIGIN OF THE HUMAN SOUL

Gonna leave this world for awhile
And I'm free, I'm free fallin'.
—Tom Petty

The mega-expansion of the Soul's desire sucked in an unimaginable amount of excess energy from Seventh Heaven. That monstrous surge roared through the Soul during the Second Bite like plugging a toaster into a nuclear power plant. It was an energy overload of such magnitude that it broke the Soul into two, creating separate male and female energies. Adam detached from Eve. These two halves fractured again, shattering into countless pieces. These shattered pieces are the origins of human souls.

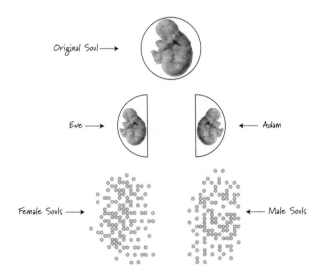

Original Soul ⟶

Eve ⟶   ⟵ Adam

Female Souls ⟶   ⟵ Male Souls

THE DESCENT INTO DEATH

The newly intensified desire of the Soul created an even greater dissimilarity between the Soul and the Light, which resulted in an increase in a greater separation due to the Law of Attraction. And that is when it happened: All these shattered sparks of souls descended into the lowest dimension of all—our physical universe.

Herein lies the secret behind the biblical phrase *The Fall of Adam*. This is also the code behind the *Expulsion from the Garden of Eden*. An increase in dissimilarity distanced the Soul from the Light, pushing it out of the Garden of Eden (the Six Dimensions) and into the most remote dimension of all—our universe.

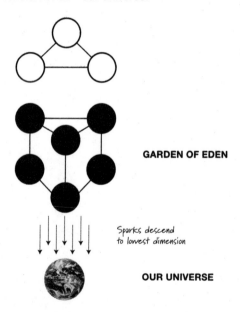

GARDEN OF EDEN

Sparks descend
to lowest dimension

OUR UNIVERSE

In this dark and distant physical realm, death was part of the landscape. And this is why the Creator told Adam and Eve they would surely die if they tasted the forbidden fruit.

BIRTH OF THE ATOM

You might say that Adam had now become atom. More specifically, the shattered sparks of Adam became the force that gave rise to the proton and all male souls. This is why protons have a positive (+) charge. Adam was the positive (+) aspect of the One Soul.

The shattered sparks of Eve became the essence of the electron and all female souls. This is why an electron has a negative charge (-). It represented the negative pole (-) in the One Soul. And, by the way, the Soul's conscious act of Resistance expressed itself as the neutron inside the atom.

Everything in our cosmos is a piece of the once unified Soul. This includes the animal, vegetable, and inanimate kingdoms. This is why all kingdoms are made up of the same raw materials: atoms. The atom contains the original forces of Creation. The atom is a microcosm of the original Creation.

> The Light (+)
> The Soul (-)
> The Act of Resistance (ø)

This is quite profound when you think about it. We have, for the first time in human history, an explanation of how and why the atom came into existence. In truth, the atom is just consciousness in material form. It was the consciousness of the Light, the Soul, and the Act of Resistance (proton, electron, and neutron) that brought about all of Creation. The only reason we might find this dazzling notion difficult to grasp is that science happened to name the positive force of consciousness a proton. If science had named this force *Light*, we would quickly grasp the profound nature of our Creation story. Likewise, if science called the electron *Soul* and named the neutron *Resistance*, Kabbalah's explanation of Creation and the nature of reality would be identical to science. The fact is they are identical. Only the names are different.

THE PART CONTAINS THE WHOLE

After the cataclysmic shattering of the Soul, it would now be left to humans (representing the largest piece of the shattered Soul) to elevate all Creation through our own transformation. In other words, each individual human being must Resist selfishness, which is nothing more than the Soul's newly intensified *Desire to Receive*. Each person has the task of completing a portion of the work that was left unfinished in Eden.

Then why do we have absolutely no recollection of any of this?

This will be explained shortly. But, in truth, nothing has really changed in terms of the Soul's original objective. The endeavor of transformation that was bound together in one mass (the One Soul) merely spread out into a big chain with many links: the individual male and female souls that compose the chain of human existence, generation after generation.

THE MEANING OF EXISTENCE

The purpose of life and the work we came here to do remains the same:

Completely resist the *Desire to Receive for the Self Alone*, and then transform it into a *Desire to Receive for the Sake of Sharing*.

Remember, the Soul did not finish resisting its desire in Eden. Instead, following the deceptive advice of the Serpent, the Soul tried to *Receive for the Sake of Sharing* **before** resisting all of its desire. That was the mistake. The Soul connected to pleasure too early. The same holds true for us in our day-to-day existence. The key to success in life is this:

You must first let go of all selfish desire so that desire has absolutely no control over you.

Once you let go *completely*, you can now receive pleasure, but this time for the purpose of sharing some of this pleasure with others. If you connect too early to Light, if there remains even a little selfish desire within you, the pleasure of the Light will overtake you, and your desire will skyrocket on that Second Bite. Or, if you just connect to pleasure selfishly, receiving without any aspect of positive sharing in your behavior, you will inevitably disconnect from the Light and wind up in darkness.

Clearly, the manner and the place in which we accomplish Resistance and Sharing have changed, but the methodology for achieving pleasure, securing fulfillment, and attracting true Light in our life remains constant:

- **Each time you resist selfish receiving, you connect to the Light.**

- **Each time you receive selfishly, you disconnect from the Light.**

MARK'S SITUATION

Our friend Mark had sex with as many women as he could, but not because he was interested in sharing. He was motivated solely by self-interest. He was not sharing; he was receiving. As Mark recalls:

> Getting a blowjob or having sex with two chicks or even having sex with my girlfriend was all about me. I never even thought about or considered the girls who I was with, beyond what I could get from them in the relationship.

Accordingly, Mark achieved momentary pleasure and Light. And then he shattered. He repeated the same mistake that he (and you and I) made in Eden.

He *received* instead of *shared*.

Spiritually and emotionally speaking, Mark then descended into the realm of death—the death of pleasure. The death of a relationship. The death of one's own happiness.

CARRIE'S SITUATION

Carrie, our computer engineer, loved three-way sex because it made **her** feel good. She was not compelled by a desire to share her love and her soul with another person. On the contrary, she was motivated by her own physical desire to "fly to the sky." She was thinking about her own erotic pleasure, not that of her partners'. The thought of another woman giving her oral sex was turning her on mentally. Even when Carrie touched her partners to give them pleasure, it wasn't true sharing. Touching and kissing others was turning Carrie on. Think of it as *sharing for the sake of receiving*, which isn't really sharing at all. It's **receiving disguised as sharing**. In other words, it was all about Carrie. As a result, her selfish receiving caused her happiness to shatter in the same way the overload of Light during the Second Bite shattered the Soul in Eden.

Carrie kept all the Light for herself, so she couldn't handle the overload. She wasn't imparting any of this energy. Consequently her opposite state from that of the Creator (Receiving as opposed to Sharing) caused her to fall into the darkness and distance herself from the Light of the 99 Percent Reality. Make no mistake: the Law of Attraction is an irrevocable one.

We now find ourselves at the end of Book Four. Let us review a summary of all we've expounded upon thus far. This model will serve as our basis for understanding sex and souls on a much more practical level.

SUMMARIZING THE WHOLE SHEBANG

THE BEGINNING

First there was Light, the essence of endless happiness.

The Light created an Infinite Soul to Receive the happiness.

This resulted in the perfect Sexual Union.

THE LAW OF ATTRACTION

Their opposing natures—Sharing versus Receiving —suddenly created separation.

The Soul, however, inherited the DNA of God, which includes the potential to Share and thus the potential to reunite.

RESISTANCE

The Soul STOPPED receiving Light in order to remove the single trait that was causing all the separation—*receiving*. This is called Resistance.

That removed 99 percent of the Light. But a residue of Light remained.

The Soul had to Resist the remaining amount of Light so there would be absolutely no Light and no Desire left.

WITHDRAWAL OF THE LIGHT

In response to the Soul Resisting the Light, the Light withdrew.

The Big Bang boomed, creating space, including our universe.

TEN CURTAINS

Ten drapes were hung up in order to create the space.

Ten dimensions were then formed out of the graduating darkness.

The ten dimensions configure as follows:
- The Upper Three, which includes Seventh Heaven
- The Middle Six Dimensions, also known as the Garden of Eden
- Our physical universe of darkness and death

THE GAME IN THE GARDEN

The One Soul dwelt in the Garden, just above our universe.

The Soul had to finish Resisting the remaining *Desire to Receive*.

Resisting all Desire would allow the Soul to completely emulate the Creator—who has no Desire at all—and become just like God.

THE ADVERSARY

- An angelic force, the Serpent, was created to challenge and prevent the Soul from Resisting its Desire to Receive.

- The existence of this Adversary served one noble purpose: To allow the Soul to truly *earn* and feel what it means to be just like God by making it an extremely difficult challenge.

- The objective of the angelic force was to trick the Soul into receiving selfishly.

THE DECEPTION

- The Adversary told the Soul it could connect to the full intensity of pleasure if it did so for the purpose of sharing. This was true, and it was accomplished through a sexual connection between the Soul and the Angel, who was really a surrogate for the Light.

- They engaged in sex. Not a problem—at first. But then, suddenly, the Soul's desire skyrocketed into extreme selfishness when it began to experience this amazing pleasure.

THE SECOND BITE

- As a result, a second connection to this pleasure proved too much for the Soul to handle. It was like plugging a lamp directly into a nuclear power plant.

ADAM & EVE

- The Soul blew its circuits. It split in two, creating male and female energies: Adam and Eve.

THE SHATTERING OF THE SOUL

- The two halves of the One Soul continued shattering into countless sparks that began raining down upon the nethermost dimension . . . our universe! These sparks included all the souls of humanity.

THE PURPOSE OF LIFE

- Individual souls must now carry out the work of transformation, which consists of eradicating selfishness from their nature and learning how to receive for the sake of sharing.

- Receiving for the Sake of Sharing is considered to be a pure act of sharing. Thus, the Soul and the Light can reunite.

There you have it: 4,000 years of comprehensive kabbalistic study, once understood only by the greatest minds in history, condensed here into a few simple points.

THE SEX-CREATION STORY CONNECTION

Why is all this so significant? This cosmology is the blueprint for human sex! It is the axiom from which all existence emerges. And it gives us a powerful formula for generating enlightenment, fulfillment, and divine sexual pleasure in our life.

How will we achieve these goals? By learning how to reconnect to Seventh Heaven and by understanding the profound relationship between what transpired up there and what unfolds down here.

BOOK FIVE

SOULS, SIN, SEDUCTION AND SEX

DOWN TO EARTH

Cosmically, we know the work of the Soul (Adam and Eve) was to resist the *Desire to Receive* and then transform it into the *Desire to Receive for the Sake of Sharing*. It is now time to get "down to Earth" and put this wisdom into effect in our daily lives by giving it a practical spin.

The Zohar tells us that our 1 Percent Illusion is a reflection of the 99 Percent Reality. Our world is a mirror of the unseen reality that exists behind the curtain. Following this line of thinking, everything we discussed in our Adam and Eve creation story must also be reflected in this earthly existence.

It is.

SOMEONE TO SHARE WITH

The shattering of the One Soul is mirrored in all the male and female souls who walk this planet, past, present, and future. This shattering created an opportunity for humanity: It gave us someone else to interact with, to share with, and to grow with, transforming ourselves in the process. By interacting with other people, our selfish desires are triggered. We now have an opportunity to resist these desires. Likewise, by interacting with others, we also have someone to share with. We can learn to *Receive for the Sake of Sharing* with the rest of the people in our lives.

All the sparks from the shattered Soul give us partners in the game of life. By relating to one another, we have both the opportunity and the means to transform ourselves from selfish people who seek only to receive into people who share and behave just like the Creator, thereby earning the mind-boggling fulfillment that is our final destiny.

SOMEONE TO PLAY AGAINST

To make this game of life challenging—just as it was in the Garden of Eden—the Adversary needs to be part of the game. After all, if Sharing were an easy task, if Resisting was an effortless act, we could never earn and grasp what it means to be like God. Logically, the Adversary needs to be a major part of this crazy game called life.

He is. You just never knew it until now.

THE ADVERSARY WITHIN

The Adversary is the ego. The Adversary is your rational mind. The Adversary is all your selfish desires. And the Adversary is your anger, insecurity, anxiety, and fear. In fact, the Adversary is every single reaction that is triggered within you by the outside world.

The Adversary is the very reason that you forgot all about your true origins and the meaning of life. The Adversary also makes you unaware, or at least doubtful of his existence.

He's good, isn't he? If you doubt the whole Creation story, it's the Adversary who is planting all this doubt in your mind. You mean you thought achieving 60 times the power of an orgasm *forever* was going to be an easy accomplishment? Fat chance. The Adversary is good at his game. He's been at it successfully now for thousands of years. The Adversary is the unseen cause behind all the conflicts and wars that have raged between sex partners, families, tribes, and nations.

FINDING YOU

The only time you find and connect to your true self is when you Resist your ego, you Resist your reactions, you Resist your selfish desires, and you Resist all of your doubts. That is when something magical happens. You connect to your soul and to the 99 Percent Reality. Resisting the Adversary is how we reunite with the Light.

Resisting the Adversary is a step-by-step process. It takes place over the course of a lifetime. We must do it in business, in our friendships, in our marriage, and in our sex life. When we finally resist the Adversary completely in every area of our life, we achieve total connection to the Light of the 99 Percent Reality.

Likewise, when a critical mass of humanity resists the Adversary completely, in every single area of life, then the entire world will achieve a total connection to the Light of the 99 Percent. All of a sudden, paradise, heaven on Earth, permanent peace, and never-ending fulfillment will be ours forever. (Of course, the Adversary will now make you doubt that promise as well.)

Kabbalah serves one single purpose. It empowers you with the awareness and tools necessary to resist and defeat the Adversary in all areas of your life. It's a lifetime of effort. The purpose of this book is to focus on achieving *heaven on Earth* in the specific area of your sex life.

HUMANITY'S RESPONSIBILITY

Clearly, the deepest desire of the human soul is to reunite with its original source, the infinite, endless Light of the 99 Percent.

This is the root of all human desire and nothing of a material nature can fulfill it. Moreover, this cosmic longing lingers throughout all existence, in all the plant and animal kingdoms, but it is only human beings who can bring about the ultimate reunification due to the size of their internal souls. With that special status comes both a promise and an obligation. The promise is that we will have the spiritual ability to develop and evolve. More than rocks, plants, or apes, we have the potential to infuse our lives with meaning and enlightenment by uprooting our negative traits and resisting selfish desires. Implicit in this promise is our unique access to the 99 Percent and the Light that can remove darkness from the landscape of human civilization.

Our essence, then, is both earthly and heavenly. We are of this world, formed from stardust. Like other living things, we eat, we sleep, and we're influenced by the fierce pull of primal instincts. But we are not just animals. We have the *free will* to choose not to react to egocentric impulses. We have the *free choice* to resist selfish desires.

Modern-day geneticists have begun unraveling and mapping the genetic codes of both humans and animals. We now know that the human DNA code is remarkably similar to that of the most highly intelligent primates, our closest evolutionary relatives. At first glance, in fact, the DNA of a human and that of a chimpanzee may look indistinguishable. But that tiny discrepancy, that 1 percent difference opens us up to an immense and mysterious universe. That 1 percent is what elevates us. It represents the ineffable human Soul and its enormous *Desire to Receive*.

When we live like animals—impulsive, reactive, guided only by self-interest—we're negating this unique gift from the Infinite. We're turning our backs on our humanity, on the cosmic promise of who we could be. Therefore, it is incumbent upon each one of us to elevate this world and reveal the sacred through our behavioral interactions, sexual connections, and spiritual transformation.

The world rises and falls on this. The job of our ego, our Adversary, is to convince us right now and every day that this is absolutely not true. Your free will allows you to reject this skepticism and realize that your kindness and proactive behavior toward your friends and enemies is the only way you can remove darkness from your life and from this world. Kindness is not about morality. Kindness is, in fact, the ultimate form of greed. It pays off for everyone.

AS ABOVE, SO BELOW

Each day, we have the opportunity to accomplish the task of resisting the Adversary through our interactions with others in business, social relationships, friendships, family ties, marriage, and, of course, through sex!

Each time an individual resists a reaction, he or she connects to the 99 Percent Reality and the **entire world** ALSO elevates and receives Light as a result of this person's effort. Likewise, each time an individual chooses to react and follow the whims of his or her own ego, a little more distance comes between that person and the Light. Now the ENTIRE world grows a bit darker.

I know what you are thinking: *Why can't we see the profound effect that our own personal behavior has upon the world?* For one reason: Because at every moment, everyone's actions are affecting the world simultaneously. This is why we cannot perceive the influence our kindness and sharing actions have upon all reality. The state of the world, the condition of human civilization, is merely the sum total of our actions. Likewise, the state of our sex life is merely the result of our behavior toward all the people in our life.

THE ADVERSARY STRIKES BACK

Usually at this juncture, the Adversary, our ego, speaks up and tells you: This is absolutely not true. The world is, in fact, random. My own actions cannot influence the entire world. I have to look out for myself in this dog-eat-dog existence.

That is just the Adversary up to his old tricks.

- He tricks you into believing that his voice is YOUR voice.

- He tricks you into believing that your behavior has no impact upon the world.

- He makes you believe that you are helpless. Insignificant. Unimportant.

Well, it's not true. In fact, your actions do not just change "a little bit" of the world. Kabbalah says your actions change the ENTIRE world. When you resist a reaction, you change the entire planet. Unfortunately, when someone else treats another human being with intolerance, he too changes the entire planet. But this makes what you do even more important.

Everything we do impacts the universe. Everything! Never forget it.

COUNTLESS CHOICES

As a result of all these shattered sparks of souls populating our world, we are faced with numerous opportunities for short-term relationships, multiple sex partners, and one-night stands. Confronted with all these choices, how does one distinguish between the fleeting pleasure of a quick fling and the deep fulfillment of a long-term relationship founded upon true love?

SOUL MATE

When the One Soul shattered into pieces like a great cosmic puzzle, every piece of the shattered male half had a corresponding puzzle piece from the fractured female aspect. Each of us has a soul mate somewhere in this world, the other piece of the puzzle. When two pieces come together in a genuine soul mate union, we are slowly rebuilding the original Soul.

Thus, when you meet your true soul mate, you feel something profoundly indescribable for the other person. Not the burst of pleasure and passion that often accompanies infatuation. Something deep. This is your perfect match, your soul mate, your other half. You fit each other completely, like two puzzle pieces that snap into place, and you are joined for all eternity.

Ultimately, from a sexual standpoint, the shattered Soul and our desire to reunite all the pieces back into one whole is the underlying cause for the particular sexual energies that emanate between people. All our sexual urges are rooted in these primordial forces of attraction, which were created when the Soul fractured in two and then shattered into many. The desire for sex is our longing to recombine into our original form.

Kabbalist Rav Berg explains the concept of soul mates as it is discussed in *The Zohar*:

> Soul mates are but two halves—male and female—of what began as a single soul in the Upper World, then divided by the hand of the Creator [the Shattering of the Soul] in preparation for the long trek through our physical world. Only when spiritual growth is accomplished and karmic debts are discharged can they come together on this plane. However, no marriage is a mistake. We must earn our other half by resisting our selfish desires. Marriage to someone other than our soul mate gives us the ability to resist reactive behavior and thus merit the other half of our soul.

THE SIGNIFICANCE OF A SIGNIFICANT OTHER

Where there is no Receiver, there can be no giving. During sex, we are given the opportunity to Share, to absorb the Light and reflect it outwards. We can't do that when we're alone. We reach our highest level of spirituality and human development in interrelationship with another.

There needs to be a space in our lives that remains open and accessible, receptive not just to another's body, but also to another's soul. It takes conscious effort to make room for the possibility of deep sexual and emotional connection. It seems easy enough. But is it? Too often we fill that space with obstacles. We clutter it . . .

With fear.
(What if no one finds me attractive? What if I'm rejected?)

With workaholism.
(I define success through my career . . . I don't have time for a relationship.)

With escapism.
(Who needs a relationship when I have crazy parties and wild flings?)

With old wounds we refuse to part with.
(Another woman/man will inevitably hurt me like she/he did.)

With the cult of materialism.
(Not yet. When I have a house/new car/more money, then I'll be happy and ready for a relationship.)

And even with excessive attachment to our pets as emotional substitutes!
(I'm not alone, I have my dog. My dog really loves me.)

Ultimately, we rise or fall together. We need companionship and we need love in order to complete ourselves and achieve our life's purpose.

That's an extremely unfashionable thing to say in our times, but there it is. Does it mean that single people are somehow lesser human beings? Of course not! A single person can be living a life distinguished by sharing and kindness and growth, while the married couple living next door might betray each other and quarrel endlessly about material things. But would that single person reach even higher levels of spiritual completeness in the context of love? The kabbalists would say yes. Our souls are in constant pursuit of reunification.

THE UPPER AND LOWER WORLD

Our physical world of desire (the 1 Percent) and the hidden dimensions of Light (the 99 Percent) are also known kabbalistically as the Lower World and the Upper World, respectively.

Adam and Eve also represent this concept of Upper and Lower World. The Upper and Lower World are expressed through male and female energies.

Male personifies the Upper World.
Female personifies the Lower World.
Male is the Light.
Female is the Soul.
Male is the rain.
Female is the Earth that receives rain and manifests life with it.
A male imparts semen.
A female receives it and manifests human life.

When male and female energies connect sexually:

The Upper and Lower Worlds connect simultaneously.

This allows the Light to flow into our lives and into our world. This is how and why we experience pleasure during sex. The Upper and Lower World relationship works in a similar fashion in our world; it is embedded into all areas of life.

When we eat a fruit:

> The fruit is the Light.
> We are the Soul, the recipient.

When the two join (through our eating), the Upper and Lower Worlds join. Hence, we feel pleasure and draw nourishment from the fruit.

When we engage in business:

> The success we seek embodies the Upper World.
> Our desire for success personifies the Lower World.

When we attain success, we have connected the Upper and Lower World and Light flows to us. This is the feeling of security, pride, and accomplishment that money often gives us.

When we eat a bar of chocolate:

> The joyous pleasure that chocolate induces is the Upper World.
> Our uncontrollable craving for chocolate corresponds to the Lower World.

When we eat chocolate, the cocoa fat produces opiates in our brain that results in pleasure; it is at that precise moment that the two Worlds unite.

Everything in life derives from either the Upper or Lower world.

Everything!

When these two worlds are joined, Light flows. Any form of pleasure that we experience is caused by a joining of the Lower and Upper World, the 1 Percent and the 99 Percent. Sex just happens to be the most powerful way to join the two worlds. Sex gives more pleasure than eating a chocolate bar—though not for everyone, unfortunately. According to a study taken in 1995, 70 percent of women would rather have chocolate than sex. Do you know why? Chocolate contains the chemical phenyl ethylamine, which mimics the brain chemistry of a person in love.

The real problem is that on a day-to-day basis, particularly with sex, we do not know how to make enduring and lasting connections between the two worlds.

THE PROBLEM OF SELFISH RECEIVING

When we try to connect to fulfillment through our ego, through self-centered desires, the two realms do not meet. We do not attain lasting Light. We get a quick fix of immediate gratification that satisfies our ego, but the two worlds quickly move away from one another. The 1 Percent and the 99 Percent grow further apart.

When this happens consistently in our lives, our world eventually becomes blanketed in darkness. The thrill of a new car disappears. The passion of sex wears off. Happiness and joy eventually cease. When we react, we have separated the 1 Percent Illusion from the 99 Percent Reality, the Upper World from the Lower World, our body from our soul. Darkness is the inevitable result (along with an increased craving for chocolate)!

Good news: There is a methodology for creating a lasting union between the 1 Percent and the 99 Percent, and it is the basis of the remainder of this book. But first . . .

THE KEY IDEAS OF BOOK FIVE

We are here to finish the work we started in the Garden of Eden, which is to transform from being selfish, reactive Receivers into proactive beings who Share.

We learn to be Sharing people by interacting with other people and Resisting self-interest.

Our Adversary in life is the Ego, our reactive nature.

Each transformation we make as individuals transforms the entire world at the same time, measure for measure.

Each of us originates from the One Soul that shattered. We each have a soul mate, the other half of our soul, with whom we seek to reunite. But this unification of two halves of one soul must be earned.

All of existence is based upon the concept of the Upper World (Light) and the Lower World (our realm of human desire). Fulfillment flows to us when these two realms unite.

BOOK SIX

HOW TO AVOID SEX WITH A SERPENT

The problem is that God gives men a brain and a penis, and only enough blood to run one at a time.
   —Robin Williams

THE ADVERSARY AT WORK

In round one of the cosmic contest, the Serpent scored a decisive blow against the Soul, resulting in the Soul falling to the canvas—our physical world. The Serpent cunningly deceived the Soul into connecting to the Light of pleasure before the Soul's selfish desire was fully expunged from its nature. This was the encoded message behind Eve taking a bite out of the apple.

Now, as we make our way through this physical existence, we do it with the Adversary temporarily attached to our nature. Our job is to lose him. Fast. But he makes it difficult. He controls 99 percent of our nature. He controls all of our thoughts. *All of them!*

THE VOICE

The Voice you hear inside your head, day in and day out, is the Adversary. The Voice broadcasts 24 hours a day. The only time you can hear your *genuine voice* is when you resist that constant loud Voice and you connect to the whispers emanating from your soul.

The Voice of the Adversary utilizes one vocabulary and one vocabulary only: Greed. Selfishness. Covetousness. Excessive self-indulgence. Insatiability. Self-interest. Keep in mind we are not talking about blatant selfishness or obvious acts of greed. The Voice is far too clever for that. Most of the time our selfishness is disguised as sharing. Our self-centeredness masquerades as goodness. We think we are helping others or sharing with friends, but in truth, we are doing it for the purpose of receiving. It could be praise, it could be honor, or it could be a feeling of self-righteousness, but there is something in it for us.

According to Kabbalah, you will know if your actions are truly acts of sharing if at first there is genuine pain, doubt, cynicism, and unwillingness before your sharing action takes place. In other words, we must give until it hurts. The pain and hurt is our clue that we are really overcoming the Adversary and his persuasive Voice. Each time we overcome the Voice, we reveal Light.

Sex is the most powerful way to reveal the Light of the Creator in this physical existence. For this reason, the Voice focuses an enormous amount of his attention in this area of our lives.

Sex is either the most wonderful and loving of human activities, or it becomes boring. Sex can also become the most violent, abusive, and terrorizing of activities. It all depends upon the degree of selfishness that is awakened in our nature; it all depends how loud and influential the Voice is.

Our selfish desire often becomes so powerful that it is like a black hole in deep space where even Light cannot escape the "gravitational pull." And the Adversary (ego) is so adept at doing its job we don't even recognize it 99 percent of the time. To quote a line of dialogue from the film *The Usual Suspects*:

> *The greatest trick the Devil ever pulled was convincing humanity that he doesn't exist.*

Replace the word *Devil* with *Ego*, and you'll begin to see the problem.

It is the ego that has also helped *Elbow God Out* of the picture in this physical realm. Our egos love to make us believe that we're the brilliant architects of our success, that we are great lovers, and that we, alone, can fulfill our partner's every need. We have no need of Light.

As the great 18th century mystic and kabbalist, Rav Israel ben Eliezer (known as, the Baal Shem Tov or the *Master of the Good Name*), once said:

Before you can find God, you must lose yourself!

Replace the word God with *great sex*, and the statement by this eminent sage still holds true!

THE DECEPTION

The Adversary prevents us from experiencing constant wild sex with our spouse. It's not someone else's fault. It's not something physical. It's not a lack of chemistry or the inevitable boredom of being with the same partner for a long period of time. Those are never the underlying reasons for disappointing sex. Each time we listen to the Voice and engage in sex through our selfish desire, we disconnect from the 99 Percent. The lamp is unplugged. The Light goes out.

When you Resist your ego, you unleash the power of your soul. And your soul is the way back to Seventh Heaven and sensational sex. However, this is easier said than done.

Resisting our *Desire to Receive* is a tremendously difficult task, because the ego is such a fierce, formidable, and fiendish opponent. And it uses the same tricks that it used in the Garden. It uses the Art of Deception! We start out with good intentions, but the moment we taste pleasure, selfishness is awakened. Pleasure overwhelms us. Good intentions turn bad. This is why Carrie's relationships self-destructed. Carrie's group of three started out pleasuring one another sexually. But it was all based on receiving pleasure, not sharing it unconditionally. As they received pleasure, they disconnected from the 99 Percent. When they lost their connection to the Light, darkness followed. They felt depressed, betrayed and dead, both spiritually and sexually speaking.

Never forget: The Adversary has the same objective as he did in Eden: Deceive the Soul (you) into selfishly receiving pleasure. The more selfish we are, the greater the separation between our souls and the Light.

How does the Adversary relate to sex?

SEXUAL THOUGHTS AND FEELINGS

As we've learned, sexual connection between two loving people is the most powerful way to reveal the Light in this world. Therefore, the Adversary directs the majority of his attention to this area. He tries to demean and defile sex as much as possible. He begins by influencing our feelings and implanting thoughts in our mind to extinguish the fires of passionate sharing that fuel a successful relationship. Instead, he fans the flames of self-interest.

Here are a few ways in which the Adversary sabotages our sex lives.

HOW THE ADVER-SARY AFFECTS MEN AND WOMEN DURING FOREPLAY:

- She desires sensual stimulation. He craves prompt penetration.

- She requests soulful titillation. He suggests intoxication.

- She wants unhurried bodily sensations. He's still trying for immediate penetration.

- She wants to touch affectionately. He wants his orgasm immediately.

- He finds lovemaking a thing of beauty. She considers it a tiring duty.

- He's hot, sexy, passionate, and wired. She's cold, cranky, disinterested, and tired.

- He wants her passion to soar on high. She accidentally thinks of another guy.

HOW THE ADVERSARY AFFECTS MEN AND WOMEN DURING SEX:

- He wants her so badly he can no longer take it. She's too tired so she decides to fake it.

- He's trying to make love erotic and slower. She can't wait to get the whole thing over.

- He's thinking about a woman at work. She's thinking that she married a jerk.

- He has more fun when he's using his hand. She can't believe this is the "promised land."

- She's finally started to feel some sensations. He's just completed his ejaculation.

HOW THE ADVER-SARY AFFECTS MEN AND WOMEN AFTER SEX:

- She wants an emotional connection. He wants to read the business section.

- She wants to talk and build rapport. He's rolled over and begun to snore.

The ego constantly compels us to engage in selfish sex and self-absorbed behavior. The result? We achieve short-term pleasure, long-term emptiness, and increased distance from the Light of happiness.

Let's examine this idea further.

DISCONNECTION: THE SECOND BITE

Emily was born in New York City. Her childhood was spent in South Orange, New Jersey. When she was eleven years old, her parents separated. Emily's brother moved with her dad in New York while Emily moved with her mom to South Florida to be with family. As a young teen in Boca Raton, Emily discovered boys. She also discovered certain desires within herself.

When I was fifteen I had a boyfriend. He always used to tell me he wanted to go all the way with me. I knew I wasn't going to sleep with him because I always had this perfect vision of how I was going to lose my virginity. This vision didn't include him. But I really got excited by rebelling and doing things I shouldn't be doing. Every day after school we would fool around in my house. We'd be totally naked and fool around in every room in the house. The shower. The closet. The kitchen. On my bed. On the couch. He would put honey on my body and lick it off. I would give him blowjobs. He would give me oral sex. I would always ask him to give me an orgasm as a way to both tease and please him and of course please myself.

Knowing that my mom could walk in any moment and catch us made it even more exciting. I wouldn't tell my friends about what I was doing because all the secretiveness turned me on.

He was always telling me he wanted to go all the way, but I refused. I felt bad about it so I did as much as I could without actually having intercourse. One day we were in the shower fooling around. One thing led to another and suddenly he was inside of me. I freaked out. I felt so violated. I had let things go too far, and now I was sorry for it. I broke up with him. I was feeling empty and gross. I didn't know what to do with myself. A few days later I started throwing up. It turned into an eating disorder and for the next four years of my life I threw up three times a day.

This is the Second Bite Syndrome. We start out with one intention, but as soon as we begin connecting to Light, we can no longer handle it. We shatter.

- Emily's intention was to tease her boyfriend and please herself without going all the way. This is the First Bite.

- The teasing and foreplay escalated into intercourse. This is the Second Bite.

- Emily underwent a meltdown. Guilt. Remorse. And finally, she developed an eating disorder. This is a reenactment of the shattering of the One Soul and the descent into darkness.

Good intentions turn sour as we succumb to the overwhelming pleasure of the moment. Then we crash. This is identical to what happened to the One Soul in the Garden of Eden. And this scenario plays itself out a billion times a day, in an endless variety of ways.

The pleasure we feel from selfish sex is real. It is genuine. The Adversary triggers these desires within us to coax us into connecting to pleasure in a receiving way, as opposed to a sharing way. For Emily, it was about <u>her</u> excitement, <u>her</u> orgasms, and <u>her</u> pleasure. Thus, her pleasure was procured for selfish reasons. This caused her to disconnect from the 99 Percent, and that's when the pleasure wears off. The thrill leaves. The rush is gone.

Emily's desire to fool around with her boyfriend was based on her receiving pleasure. She loved the excitement of doing naughty things, behavior that was considered forbidden. She loved rebellion. Once she tasted the pleasure of rebellion, the Second Bite occurred and she found herself in a shower having intercourse with someone she didn't want to have intercourse with.

The Second Bite syndrome is why we feel so down after engaging in selfish behavior, why we crash after getting high from drugs, why our excitement eventually dissipates after buying a new car or new clothes. The gratification was not created through our own proactive efforts to share. It was motivated by our ego—the one and only Adversary. Consequently, the pleasure is powerful for the moment, but then the shattering reoccurs and darkness descends upon us.

THE DANGER OF DIRECT CONNEC-TIONS

What's really happening in our lives—kabbalistically—when we succumb to the temptations of ego, when we engage in selfish actions, self-centered thoughts, and self-indulgent behavior? Earlier we said that this is a re-enactment of the Soul's connection to too much energy when it connected to Seventh Heaven. Let's bring this idea down to our world and make it more practical.

Consider a battery. A battery has both a positive and negative pole. If we attach a strand of wire to both ends of the battery—directly connecting the positive (+) and negative (-) poles-what happens? The battery gradually loses all energy. The direct connection between positive and negative causes a power drain. This is called a short circuit.

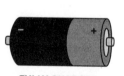

FULLY CHARGED

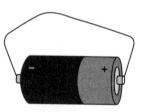

POWER DRAIN

SEXUAL POWER DRAIN

The battery is a great metaphor for human sexual relationships.

- The positive pole of a battery corresponds to sexual pleasure and the 99 Percent.

- The negative pole corresponds to the human desire for sex.

When we engage in selfish sex, Desire (-) and Pleasure (+) connect directly. This is a short circuit. Our relationship begins to experience a power drain. Sexual energy diminishes. Erotic passion slowly dissipates. We're gradually depleting our relationship of Light. This is why our relationships eventually lose their fire. A meltdown is underway. As a result, our desire for sex with the same person begins to wane.

What are we to do? How do we take control over our lives, thoughts, and desires? How do we distinguish between desires born of the ego and desires arising from our soul? How do we battle these thoughts, urges, and impulses implanted within us by our fiendish Adversary? How do we prevent those delicious, delectable, but highly dangerous direct connections to Light?

THE POWER OF RESISTANCE

We've discussed a powerful technique for keeping the Adversary from controlling our lives. Kabbalah calls it *Resistance*. It means stopping our reactive impulses and selfish receiving.

Although this action can be expressed in a brief sentence, accomplishing it requires almost superhuman willpower and self-restraint. It is *easier said than done* because the influence of our ego is so powerful.

Let's examine Resistance further.

RESISTANCE IN OUR WORLD

We've learned that the Soul *stopped* receiving the Light in order to remove the one trait (Receiving) that was creating separation between the Light and Soul. The Creator complied and withdrew the Light.

This act of Resistance is now a universal law of our universe.

In other words, Light—both spiritual and physical—can no longer be revealed unless Resistance is at work. Understanding this kabbalistic principle is the key to great sex.

There are two kinds of Resistance in our world: *Voluntary Resistance* and *Involuntary Resistance*. Let's first examine Involuntary Resistance and see how it shows up in the electrical energy and physical sunlight in our world.

INVOLUNTARY RESISTANCE

The Earth floats in the blackness of space while the sun shines its rays upon her. Why is there darkness all around the Earth? Why is it black between the Earth and the sun if the sun's rays are streaming through space?

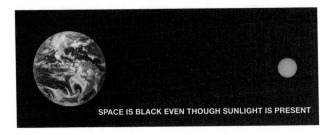

SPACE IS BLACK EVEN THOUGH SUNLIGHT IS PRESENT

The reason is that there is no resistance; no reflection is taking place in those empty areas of space. Sunlight remains invisible to the naked eye until it strikes a physical object—planet Earth—where it is then reflected.

Guess what? This act of reflection is *Resistance*! The object resists the Light. It pushes it away and in doing so, rays of sunlight suddenly shine.

Space is dark, even though the sun's photons are everywhere, because nothing in the vacuum of space is resisting the sunbeams. On Earth, the atmosphere and the physical Earth reflect, resist, and thus reveal the light of the sun. There is no choice in the matter. Physical objects naturally resist rays of light. For this reason, we call it *Involuntary Resistance*.

Consider hearing. Sound is not heard until the eardrum *resists* waves and transforms it into a sound for us to process. The light of hearing shines only through Resistance.

THE LIGHT BULB

A light bulb has both a positive and a negative pole. Separating the two is a filament, which creates resistance by stopping the free flow of electrical energy traveling between the positive and negative poles. It prevents a direct connection. Resistance is responsible for the illumination of the bulb.

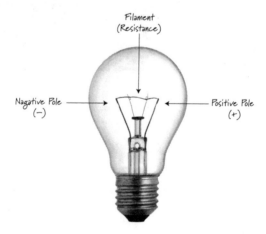

When the filament breaks, the positive pole connects **directly** with the negative pole, causing a short circuit. There is a temporary flash of light followed by darkness and a worn-out bulb. You've seen this happen when a bulb has burned out in your home. The sudden flash is brilliant but short-lived.

The filament is a natural resistor of electricity, thus we also refer to this as *Involuntary Resistance*.

Resistance also plays a role in the physiology of sex.

RESISTANCE AND THE PHYSIOLOGY OF AN ERECTION

According to Kabbalah, blood is the link between the body and soul, which is why blood has both white and red cells. The color white denotes the 99 Percent Reality of Sharing, and contains all the colors of the rainbow. It is whole. Complete. It represents absolute Sharing. White blood cells, therefore, denote the sharing aspect of the soul.

The color red corresponds to the 1 Percent Illusion. This is why red is the lowest frequency in the color spectrum. Red blood cells correspond to the body's *Desire to Receive*. Blood contains **both** aspects of the Upper and Lower worlds, the Divine and the human, the body and the soul.

Blood, therefore, represents the potential to *unify both realms!*

AN ERECTION

During sexual activity, a man's erection is generated by blood flowing into the penis. This flow of blood causes enlargement and elevation of the reproductive organ. The erection and elevation indicate the ascension into the 99 Percent Reality and the potential and promise that it holds for us.

Physically, the erection is achieved through Resistance.

- The male reproductive organ, in this instance, corresponds to the receiving aspect of the Soul. The penis becomes a Receiver.

- Blood flowing into the reproductive organ corresponds to the sharing aspect of the Light.

As blood fills the sexual organ (Light filling Soul), there is a temporary reduction in the volume of blood leaving the penis. How? Through the power of Resistance!

The veins leading from the reproductive organ have valves that *resist* the outflow of blood. Resistance traps the blood in the organ, causing it to become erect.

The male sexual organ now resides in Seventh Heaven and in our Lower World *at the same time*. It is our link between the physical and spiritual, and for this reason it generates tremendous pleasure for men and women in this earthly realm. For this reason, it has the Godlike power to help bring life into existence.

The female sexual organ—and more specifically the clitoris, which is responsible for a huge amount of the pleasure women experience during sex—also operates on the principle of Resistance. The clitoris is made of the same erectile tissue as the penis, and when aroused, it fills with blood. Once again, the outflow of blood is resisted until the woman achieves orgasm. In both sexes, we see that the key ingredient to sexual pleasure is Resistance.

FRICTION

Physics is like sex: sure, it may give some practical results,
but that's not why we do it.
　—Richard P. Feynman

Friction is a big part of sex. Two lovers locked in embrace caress one another. The friction created by two bodies in motion generates sparks of passion. In physics and in sex, friction is created through Resistance.

In elementary physics, energy is transformed into another form when it encounters Resistance. Consider the light bulb. Because the bulb's filament resists invisible electricity, the current is then transformed into visible glowing photons of light. The invisible becomes visible **after Resistance**.

Likewise, when a hand creates friction by caressing and touching the human body, the imperceptible Light of the Creator is then transformed into perceptible sexual energy and pleasure. These are all examples of Involuntary Resistance.

There is another form of Resistance and it is the absolute, irrefutable key to generating great sex.

VOLUNTARY RESISTANCE

To keep love alive, to keep passion aflame, the kabbalists revealed the concept of *Voluntary Resistance*. This form of Resistance corresponds to the act of Resistance the Soul performed when it was initially created.

Originally, the Soul Resisted the direct Light flowing from the Creator so that it would no longer be in an opposite state, stuck in a mode of receiving. This was the voluntary choice of the Soul.

Kabbalah also calls this . . .

FREE WILL

In addition to the physical resistance that occurs inside a light bulb, there is a non-material form of resistance that exists in the mind. It's called free will. We use it when we **resist our egocentric desires**.

A human being is endowed with the mental faculties to distinguish between good and evil, between selfish reactive behavior and sharing proactive behavior. Coupled with this ability to recognize these differences is our freedom to choose between them. In behavioral terms, we have the opportunity to opt for the selfish *Desire to Receive* motivated by primal lusts, or we can elect *not* to respond to self-centered impulses.

Simply put:

> *Do I think only about myself during the heat of passion or do I resist the urge and take my partner's needs into consideration first? Do I cheat on my partner to satisfy my own desire, or do I take my partner's feelings into consideration and Resist?*

According to Kabbalah, if we emulate the filament in a bulb and resist selfish desires—both in and out of the bedroom—we crank out sexual energy. This Lights up our relationship.

FORGET ABOUT MORALS

Make no mistake: It's not about moral values. It's not about honorable behavior. Nor is it about a noble code of religious conduct and scruples. Not at all! Rather, it's about: *What's in it for me?* But now we're looking below the surface, where what's in it for you happens to coincide with what's in it for everyone else.

Enlightened self-interest is our only motivation. Kabbalah is not about giving something up for some abstract spiritual ideal. Kabbalah is about learning how to have it all. When we resist the desire for immediate but short-term gratification, it's for one reason and one reason only—to attain greater pleasure over the long term! It's about turning on the Light in our life and keeping it on.

Following this kabbalistic principle, when we are in the grip of ego, self-centeredness, and receiving for its own reward, we feel passion and excitement for a brief moment when we touch Seventh Heaven during orgasm—and then we crash. Sexual energy starts to seep out of our relationship. The sexual power drain in our relationship is underway.

Every aspect of your life offers you the opportunity to apply Resistance:

- how you treat your partner in your daily life;

- how you treat your friends and your foes;

- how you react to life's obstacles and challenges; and

- how you treat people in business.

In all of the above scenarios, you have free will to either resist or not resist an egocentric response. The key to great sex—and great life—is this:

The more Resistance we apply, the more Light we generate.

The Light generated by Resistance automatically illuminates our sexual relationships. To the degree that we transform our behavior toward our partner through Resistance, sexual excitement flows into the relationship. And when we apply Resistance in our dealings with family, friends, and foes, even more passion will flow into our sexual relationships.

APPLYING RESIS-
TANCE IN SEX

Remember Michael? Michael admits that he was so consumed in his own desires he neglected the needs of his wife Meredith.

> It never dawned on me to even consider her needs. I was totally self-absorbed with my own desires. I was blinded. I did not recognize the foolishness of my actions. I was a puppet on a string. After a lot of pain, I eventually realized that my ego was pulling the strings the whole time. Before studying Kabbalah, I had no idea the ego was a separate force that constantly sabotaged my life. I focused on immediate gratification, never once connecting the chaos in my life to my own behavior. I blamed everything and everyone but myself.

The Adversary constantly plagues our minds with doubts concerning the existence of the Light and the purpose of life. The Adversary even implants doubts about the wisdom of this book. And make no mistake: the ego will even summon forth doubts about the validity of the last two statements!

Michael adds:

> When I finally realized that there was a real force battling inside of me, I stopped taking my selfishness so seriously. I saw that negative thoughts and desires didn't really belong to me. I began to understand that it was the Adversary who was convincing me that my selfish thoughts were real. It wasn't easy. It still isn't.

When I began resisting my ego, I saw results. I saw miracles take place. Literally. Regarding sex, it used to be how great I could make my orgasm. I would fantasize about other girls while making love to my wife. I would fantasize about her having sex with other men during intercourse to arouse myself. I started blocking those thoughts. I focused my attention on my wife, thinking about sharing with her, considering her needs first. I also stopped flirting with other women. I wanted to see what would happen in my marriage. I tried some other kabbalistic tools, as well. I never would have believed the results if I hadn't experienced them firsthand. After 17 years of marriage, our sex life went to a whole new level. Passion. Excitement. Chemistry. Its not mind-blowing sex every time, but the difference is like night and day.

Michael's insights are extremely important. He realized that the Adversary was not actually part of his own essence and being. This is a hugely important realization that often takes people years to grasp. In fact, you may be having difficulty right now accepting the idea that the loud Voice and those constant impulses that flood your mind do not really belong to you. But it's true. The Adversary plants those impulses, desires, and thoughts within you. And he even goes one step further by implanting doubts about his own existence and his role. He does this for one reason: *So that you remain ignorant of his existence, which leaves him in full control over your life.*

Until we truly understand that the Adversary is real, and that he was created to test us and challenge us in the cleverest ways possible, we will never find the motivation to fight him, resist him, and transform our sex lives into something profound and passionate. Just keep reminding yourself that that negative thought, doubt, and selfish urge is not who you really are. We can feel this truth in the depth of our souls simply by applying resistance. Resist the thought. Resist the urge. Resist the selfish impulse. Then watch what happens. The proof lies in your own experience.

TOOLS OF THE TRADE

Please be forewarned: The following are merely tools designed to help you connect to Energy. You are free to use all of them, some of them or none of them. This is not, absolutely not, an all-or-nothing situation. Just as we learned from our example of the light bulb, the more Resistance you apply, the more you can increase the wattage of your sex life. There's no right or wrong involved.

And always remember:

- No one has the right to tell you how many tools to incorporate in your life.

- No one has the right to tell you what *short circuits* to avoid.

- No one has the right to judge you.

- No one has the right to tell you that this Kabbalah stuff really works, especially the author. It's up to you to determine that on your own.

We are all sparks of the Divine. Each one of us is sacred, and we are all equally loved by the Creator, according to Kabbalah. Thus, our free will and personal choices in life must be respected and honored.

There is one more important piece of wisdom that we need to remember in order to activate and "switch on" all these kabbalistic tools . . .

THE POWER OF KNOWLEDGE

Information is *not* power. Knowledge is power. This insight is found in a biblical verse that has confounded scholars, rabbis, and priests for thousands of years, even to this very day. The biblical verse refers to Adam and Eve and the birth of Cain. Found in Genesis, it states:

Adam knew Eve his wife, and she bore Cain.

The kabbalists asks the question: Why would The Bible use the word "knew" to imply a sexual act between a man and a woman? Why not use the word intercourse? Who can recall an instance where a woman became pregnant simply by knowing a man?

This strange biblical verse is really just a code:

Adam is a code for the 99 Percent Reality.

Eve is a code for our physical world, the 1 Percent Illusion of unsatisfying sex.

Knew is a code for the concept of having knowledge.

It works like this: When you want to connect the two worlds so that Light will flow into your life, you must possess *kabbalistic knowledge* as to how and why things work in the physical and spiritual realms. In other words, blind faith won't cut it. Knowledge is how one makes a connection to the 99 Percent. According to Kabbalah, the wrong information or just plain ignorance will always keep you in the dark. Correct spiritual knowledge connects you to Light. Knowledge is the link. Intercourse between the 1 Percent and the 99 Percent takes place only when knowledge pervades our consciousness. In other words,

- **You have to know all about the existence of the 99 Percent in order to connect to it.**

- **You have to know how and why sex came into existence in order to experience great sex.**

- **You have to know about the existence of the Adversary in order to destroy it.**

Never underrate the power of kabbalistic knowledge. It is nothing like learning geography or history, subjects which can make you more educated but still just represent information. Kabbalistic knowledge is the actual Light itself. It is the substance of spiritual energy. When that knowledge becomes part of your being, part of your essence, there is less darkness inside of you.

SEXUAL SHORT CIRCUITS

Let's revisit the Garden of Eden for a moment and recall the original showdown between the Soul and the Serpent. The goal of the Soul while in the Garden was to Resist its Desire to Receive 100 percent. The Serpent, however, deceived the Soul into "eating" from the Tree of Knowledge prematurely.

As we've seen, the Serpent did this by hiding deception behind a thin veil of truth. The Serpent told the Soul it could connect to Seventh Heaven if it did so with the intent to *Receive for the Sake of Sharing* with the Creator. This was true. The Serpent told the Soul that if it stopped receiving forever, the Soul would wind up empty. The Light can be expressed only if there is a bona fide desire to receive Light. Hence, the Serpent told the Soul, that the ultimate objective was actually to receive, but only for the purpose of sharing. This way the Soul could receive and share at the same time. This was true. But what the Serpent failed to mention was that the Soul had to first eradicate and resist ALL *Desire to Receive* before it attempted to *Receive for the Sake of Sharing*.

The Soul had never tasted the pleasure of Seventh Heaven, so it was easy to commit to receiving for the sake of sharing before taking a bite. Thus the First Bite was pure. But the little bit of desire that remained inside the Soul could not handle the intensity of pleasure. After the First Bite, the Soul's desire skyrocketed into the stratosphere. Therefore, on the Second Bite, the Soul's desire was out of control and the Soul began receiving selfishly. This caused a system overload and, in turn, the shattering of the Soul into a gazillion pieces.

Let's call this strategy of the Adversary—*The Deception*.

PLEASURE AND POISON

The Adversary's artful act of deception reenacts in our physical world in many ways. The Adversary hides harm behind pleasure. The great Kabbalist Rav Ashlag provides an illustration:

If a man has a wound on his body and it itches him continually, constantly begging to be scratched, the act of scratching brings the man great reward in the form of pleasure. However, there is a drop of "the poison of death" mixed in with the pleasure (just as the Serpent coated his lie with a layer of truth in the Garden).

If the person scratching the wound does not take control over his impulses and he continues to pay off these persistent pangs to be scratched, his very payments will serve to increase his debt. Namely, in proportion to the pleasure he attains by furiously scratching and receiving pleasure, his wound grows proportionately larger. His pleasure will soon turn into pain. When a wound begins to heal, a new demand to be scratched usually arises and the itch intensifies. If a man is still not able to control his impulses and he persists in paying off this nagging demand by scratching the wound, the wound worsens, eventually bringing a drop of bitterness, which will poison all of his blood. Thus, the man becomes gravely ill or even dies as a direct result of the pleasure that he originally gave himself. This is because it was limited pleasure rooted in immediate gratification.

This important concept calls for one more example:

THE MAGIC POTION

Suppose the Adversary concocted a magic potion that aroused untold pleasure with every sip. Into this blissful concoction, however, the Adversary injected a single drop of poisonous venom that was undetectable to our taste buds. When you drink the magic tonic, you're overwhelmed with pleasure. But, at the same time, you're completely unaware of the deadly drops that have just entered your system. Each sip, each new cup of bliss that you ingest, slowly dims the Light of your soul. Eventually, the very pleasure you receive brings your death.

> *The pleasure derived from egocentric behavior is that toxic tonic.*

Receiving pleasure directly for oneself alone and instinctively reacting to everything and everyone around us is a pleasurable but poisonous potion that brings us instant gratification along with a drop of death with every sip. What dies is the Light of our soul. What dies is our sex life.

THE POWER OF LIGHT

Light is the fuel of sexual energy. Light is also the force of financial prosperity, the essence of enlightenment, the stuff of serenity, the power of peace of mind, the substance of stillness, the energy that is our immune system. When the Light is dimmed, it has an adverse effect on our business, health, emotional stability, and our sexual relationships. The key to sexual pleasure and a life of fulfillment is to avoid the drink of death, and not to scratch the itch of affliction.

But make no mistake, this is a difficult task to achieve because the Adversary brings us trays of luscious cocktails all day long. He mercilessly tickles our ego so that it begs to be scratched all the time, in every part of our lives. The Serpent—our ego and Adversary—attempts to seduce us into Second Bites by tricking us into taking the First Bite with good and pure intentions. Selfish pleasure, or 1 Percent Sex, brings along with it a hidden fire extinguisher that gradually snuffs out the Light in our sex lives.

THE BIG QUESTION

Now comes the big question: What do the kabbalists classify as 1 Percent Sex? And how do we incorporate the technique of Resistance to avoid it? Any kind of sex that is based upon receiving pleasure selfishly without intent to merge with another person's soul in a purely sharing and loving fashion, is 1 Percent Sex.

Experiences of 1 Percent Sex include:

- thinking about your own pleasure before your partner's;

- for a male, coming to orgasm before your partner;

- flirting with someone other than your mate;

- having extramarital affairs;

- having sex during a woman's menstrual cycle;

- masturbating;

- titillating yourself with pornography; and

- thinking of someone else while making love to your partner.

DUMP MORALITY

If electricity comes from electrons, does that mean that morality comes from morons?
—Unknown

Let me remind you that the items in our 1 Percent Sex list have nothing—absolutely nothing at all—to do with morality, guilt, or religious principles. Kabbalah is all about energy flow, the physics of spirituality, and methodologies for generating megawatts of sexual power. Toss morality and ethical behavior out the window; flush shame and guilt down the toilet; stuff "religious" principles into the trash compactor. Kabbalah has nothing to do with these concepts.

If 1 Percent Sex delivered a lasting connection to pleasure, the kabbalist would be the first in line for it. But 1 Percent Sex doesn't do the trick.

All of which brings us to our seventh and final chapter.

THE KEY IDEAS OF BOOK SIX

The Adversary is part of our nature, though we don't recognize it most of the time.

The Adversary draws us into behaving selfishly by seducing us with immediate pleasure and instant gratification.

Receiving pleasure selfishly is like a direct connection between negative and positive poles in a battery. It causes a short circuit and power drain.

Resistance is the key to prevent direct connections. It turns on the Light of sexual energy.

Resistance works like a filament in a light bulb. It resists the energy, and thus the energy is transformed into Light.

Free will allows us to choose between resisting selfish receiving, or not resisting it.

Knowledge is the link connecting us to the 99 Percent Reality of Light.

Kabbalistic wisdom and tools are not founded upon morals. They are founded upon enlightened self-interest.

BOOK SEVEN

KABBALISTIC TOOLS FOR ENHANCED SEXUAL PLEASURE

RESISTING MALE MASTURBATION

Male masturbation involves stimulating the penis to produce pleasure through ejaculation. It feels great. It's a quick thrill. It produces pleasure. Nonetheless, it is a direct connection between desire (-) and pleasure (+). This direct connection causes a short circuit.

Masturbation depletes our relationships of sexual energy. It drains us of the sexual power we need in the future. This is one reason why the excitement wanes in our relationships. If you apply Resistance and refrain from self-pleasuring, with the sole intent to connect to Light, sexual energy builds back up. Not only does it build back up, it actually multiplies!

FACT FROM FICTION

No, you won't go blind or grow hair on your palms. These superstitions just distract us from what's really going on.

First of all, masturbation is not a sharing action. It gratifies only 1 percent of our being—the ego. One person is benefiting. There is no imparting pleasure to someone else. This is *Desire to Receive for the Self Alone*. This kind of receiving creates separation between you and the Light of the 99 Percent. It violates the Law of Attraction.

Secondly, everything in our world is merely a shadow, a reflection of something in the 99 Percent Reality. Semen is the closest substance on Earth to Light because semen has the power to create life.

And it generates wild pleasure in the process. Creation and pleasure are essential attributes of the Light.

When semen is produced but not used to share pleasure or procreate, the powerful energy within the semen is left out in the open in this physical world like raw, naked energy. This gives the Adversary an opportunity to capture this force and use it to strengthen himself. The Adversary has no Light or power of his own. The only Light and strength he gets is what we hand over to him. Each time we react to our ego, we strengthen the Adversary. When semen, the most powerful substance on Earth, is not harnessed for a positive purpose, the Adversary hijacks this power. How?

SAFEGUARDING ENERGY

Electricity must be protected by a cable in order for us to harness it in a safe way. Nuclear energy is concealed inside the atom. If the atom is split and energy is released, it causes unimaginable destruction. If a high-voltage wire gets exposed and dangles in the streets and someone touches it, the raw naked energy can kill in an instant. The atom and the cable act like a vessel that safely contains and conceals the energy.

According to Kabbalah, semen must also have a vessel in order for it to be safely harnessed in our lives. A sharing and loving *intention* is the vessel that safely holds and conceals the Light embodied by the male's semen. Darkness cannot coexist with Light; therefore, an intention of sharing disarms the adversary. When there is no vessel, the Adversary becomes an even stronger presence in your life. And that means more misfortune is created. Any time semen is not contained in a vessel, the Adversary swoops in and uses it to generate misfortune. Naturally, when things just happen to go wrong in your life, you pass it off as random chaos. But any chaos, depression, anxiety, or pain we experience is the result of the Adversary capturing the Light that we hand over to him, leaving us in darkness. And don't forget: treating your spouse, a friend, or a foe with anything less than human dignity also empowers the Adversary. Wasting the Life Force called semen is just one way—the most powerful way—to strengthen this formidable Opponent.

However, when the semen—the Light—is used for sharing purposes, you draw down tremendous forces of Light for yourself and the world. The Adversary misses out on a meal. He grows weaker. The world becomes brighter as the union between a couple creates union between our world and the Upper World. Remember, as above, so below!

A WORD ABOUT FEMALE MASTURBATION

According to Kabbalah, masturbation by a woman does not wreak the same spiritual havoc that male masturbation causes. No sperm is left exposed when a woman masturbates. For this reason, it is not considered to be a short circuit.

On the other hand, female masturbation does not create new Light. In other words, it is not a sharing act. It pleasures only 1 percent of our being—our ego. It is self-gratification. Any action that is not designed to generate Light through sharing with a partner is considered to be a wasted action and therefore 1 Percent Sex. You and your soul stay stuck in the 1 Percent Illusion through 1 Percent Sex. You cannot elevate your life into the 99 Percent Reality through 1 Percent Sex.

For this reason, it is perhaps advantageous for women to refrain. The idea here is not to be giving something up, but rather to infuse your relationship (or future relationship) with more Light and sexual energy. If you are single, the more Light you generate in your life, the more quickly you will attract your true soul mate.

TOOLS TO HELP US RESIST

Resisting masturbation is often difficult. Individuals must do what works for them if they feel inclined to practice this technique and test-drive the teachings of Kabbalah.

To help us, the ancient kabbalists provided tools some 2,000 years ago that give us the power and strength to perform Resistance in the areas in which we choose. These tools include the ancient books of *The Zohar*.

THE POWER OF
THE ZOHAR

The Zohar is written in the ancient language of Aramaic, but you do not need to understand Aramaic when using *The Zohar* as a tool for meditation. *The Zohar* is not merely a book to read and study. In fact, *The Zohar* is not really a "book" at all in the conventional sense. To the kabbalists, *The Zohar* is a cable, an antenna, a vital connection to the immense Force and Light of the 99 Percent Reality.

Here's how it works:

The Zohar is filled with passages that reveal profound secrets about life, tackling topics that range from sex to healing. But make no mistake, *The Zohar* is not merely imparting pearls of wisdom to the reader. Far from it. *The Zohar* is also actually radiating the energy of the solution to the particular problems it is addressing. This is the real secret of *The Zohar*. This is its great mystery. That is what 99 percent of the scholars who have tried to study Kabbalah have never grasped or understood.

The Zohar delivers the cure! *The Zohar* provides the solution. *The Zohar* causes change to take place. For instance, if a specific verse speaks about heart disease, then that very same verse also radiates the energy that heals heart disease. Pretty amazing!

So how do we harness this energy? We do it through our eyes and through meditation.

For example, there are potent meditative passages inside *The Zohar* that empower us with the strength to perform Resistance in every area of our life. Below you will find a *Zohar* passage that deals with masturbation and the dangers of leaving semen exposed.

These ancient Aramaic verses dissolve unwanted desires from our consciousness. They also destroy the nasty negative forces that were aroused from previous sexual short circuits. And they help recharge our batteries.

Meditating upon the following passage of *Zohar* infuses you with the power to resist masturbation. You can either quickly scan the Aramaic letters with your eyes for a minute or two, or meditate intensely upon this passage for five to ten minutes. Both approaches work. The key to activating this Resistance power within you is your desire to achieve a specific goal and connect to the 99 Percent. The stronger your conviction, the more powerful the results will be.

MEDITATION

394. כִּי רַבָּה רָעַת הָאָדָם. כָּל בִּישִׁין הֲווֹ עָבְדֵי, וְלָא אִשְׁתְּלִים חוֹבַיְיהוּ, עַד דַּהֲווֹ אוֹשְׁדִין דָּמִין לְמַגָּנָא עַל אַרְעָא. וּמָאן אִינוּן. דַּהֲווֹ מְחַבְּלִין אָרְחַיְיהוּ עַל אַרְעָא. הה״ד רַק רַע כָּל הַיּוֹם. כְּתִיב הָכָא רַק רַע, וּכְתִיב הָתָם וַיְהִי עֵר בְּכוֹר יְהוּדָה רַע בְּעֵינֵי ה׳.

RESISTING ADULTEROUS THOUGHTS

During the heat of passion, sometimes even before the sparks begin to fly, it is not unusual to suddenly think of another person who you find attractive. Immediately, our "arousal meter" jumps into the red zone, making it difficult to resist these enticing thoughts, which often build up their own sexual energy. However, the passion and pleasure we gain is a short circuit. We achieve an intense burst of direct Light followed by darkness. It's like draping cloth over a lamp. Each thought dims the Light. Eventually it is extinguished.

THE ORIGIN OF ADULTEROUS THOUGHTS

The Adversary implants these thoughts in our minds. In fact, the Adversary, like the original Soul, has two aspects: male and female.

- The male aspect is known by the code term (do not pronounce this name) *Samael*.

- The female aspect is known by the code term (do not pronounce this name) *Lilit*.

The force called *Lilit* targets men, while the force known as *Samael* targets women. These are actual negative entities that battle us all the time, and will even implant cynicism in your mind to hide their existence. Their sole objective is to deceive us into short-circuiting through 1 Percent Sex.

Why? They receive all the Light that is generated through 1 Percent Sex. That is how they sustain their existence. That is how they increase their power. All you get is a short-term spark of pleasure. It feels great for the moment, but in the long term it drains sexual energy from your relationships. You are then forced to masturbate again or think of other people while making love to your partner because you feel the increased emptiness. You're forced to seek out bigger sparks of energy. Like Mark, you have to keep escalating your sexual adventures just to recapture the pleasure you lost. One partner can no longer do it for you. Now you need two partners at the same time. Or you have to have sex with drugs.

RECLAIMING CONTROL OF YOUR THOUGHTS

These two aspects of the Adversary are very familiar to you. For instance, when you know something is good for you, it is the little voice inside you that says, "Put it off till Monday." When you know something is bad for you, it is the voice that says, "Do it anyway."

When you find yourself getting aroused by imagining your partner as someone else, pause for a moment and de-arouse yourself. Let the feelings go. Start over with the intent to share with your spouse. This action will ensure that all the Light goes to you and your partner, not to the Adversary.

As you continue resisting these thoughts, you will gradually begin to recharge the battery in your relationship. Step by step, you will feel a renewed sense of fire and desire for your partner. All the years of short circuits and power drains can be erased. Just remember, it takes time to recharge a battery that has been drained over the years.

TOOLS TO CONTROL THOUGHTS

In addition to meditative technologies, Kabbalah also offers verbal tools that arouse positive forces of energy. The following Aramaic text can either be recited or visually scanned before a couple engages in sexual intercourse. This literally keeps the Adversary out of your bedroom and negative thoughts out of your head. And it will absolutely prevent any negative forces from capturing Light that is generated during your moments of intimacy.

MEDITATION

עֲטִיפָא בְּקִטְפָא אִזְדַּמְּנַת, שָׁאֲרֵי שָׁאֲרֵי, לָא תְּעוֹל וְלָא תִּנְפּוֹק,
לָא דִּידָךְ וְלָא בְּעַדְבָּךְ. תּוּב תּוּב, יַמָּא אִתְרְגִישָׁא, גַּלְגַּלוֹי לִיךְ קָרָאן,
בְּחוּלָקָא קַדִּישָׁא אֲחִידְנָא, בִּקְדוּשָׁה דְּמַלְכָּא אִתְעַטַּפְנָא.

A TRANSLITERATION OF THE ABOVE BLESSING
(read left to right)

Atifa bekitfa izdamnat, sharei, sharei, la ta'ol ve la tinpok, la didach, ve la be'adbach. Tuv, tuv yama etragisha, galgaloyi li'ach karan, bechulaka kadisha achidna, bekedusha demalka ite'atafena.

RESISTING NEGATIVE SEXUAL THOUGHTS AND THE GUILT THEY AROUSE

All negative thoughts come from the Adversary. All of them! No matter how unique these thoughts seem to be, do not take ownership of them. They do not originate from your true essence and being. They are implanted within you. The only time we create darkness in our lives is when we believe those thoughts are our own and we act upon them. When we recognize that these thoughts are the work of the Adversary, and we gently resist and push them away, we bring Light into the world. Too often, we feel guilty, weird, depressed, worried, or shameful because we have unusual sexual thoughts. Not any longer. Let go of those negative and useless feelings and find true freedom. Now you know that you are not weird. You are not twisted. You are not strange. You are not crazy. You are not abnormal. You are a wonderful human being, a genuine spark of the Creator who came to this world to discover this truth and to battle the Adversary by not accepting his thoughts as your own.

TOOLS TO CONTROL THOUGHTS

This next ancient meditation eradicates all obsessive thoughts, negative sexual thoughts, or thoughts that induce anxiety and fear. It stops them dead in their tracks.

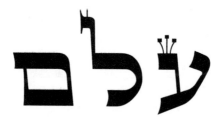

RESISTING PORNOGRAPHY

When we become aroused by pornography, all the Light we generate goes to the Adversary because we are in a state of receiving. The Law of Attractions kicks in, and we move away from the 99 Percent Reality. Therefore, we feel pleasure at first, but then darkness overcomes us as we increase our separation from the Light. This is the why porn eventually stops turning us on. We have magnified our disconnection from the 99 Percent and it becomes harder to connect to pleasure. Now we need harder porn to generate excitement, and we're caught in a vicious cycle. Our distance from the 99 Percent affects all of our relationships. Passion diminishes. Sexual energy weakens.

RESISTING FLIRTING

There are many ways to flirt: at the office, anonymously in a chat room, via phone sex, or with your spouse's best friend. We do it with words. We do it with our hands. We do it with our lips.

Flirting is 1 Percent Sex. There is no intent to share or build a loving relationship with another person. You are using the other person to simply fulfill your own desire. It's self-gratification. Receiving. Again, we have a direct connection to energy.

- Your desire to flirt is the negative (-) charge.

- The pleasure generated is the positive charge (+).

You receive a spark of Light followed by a short circuit and darkness. This darkness is what kills the fire in an existing relationship.

RESISTING CHEATING

During the Middle Ages in France, an unfaithful wife was forced to chase a chicken through town naked. In ancient Rome, two-timing women were condemned to death. Asiatic Huns castrated adulterous males.

According to Kabbalah, punishments will never curb adultery. Punishments are a fanatical response to an age-old phenomenon, and as such are considered abusive, intolerant behavior.

What will help a person refrain from adultery is pure, unadulterated greed. *Greed*? Yes, greed! The problem with cheating on a partner is our lack of knowledge concerning the true spiritual consequences. And we've lost sight of the immense payoff that comes with remaining faithful.

THE WEAPON OF TIME

The Adversary is not stupid. He is shrewd. Cunning. What does he do? He uses time to throw you for a loop. How? *Time* is used to delay the consequences of your actions, to obscure the power of cause and effect. The consequences of our actions appear at a later date. It's a clever tactic. Why? The passage of time makes you forget the original cause. You never detect the correlation between the chaos in your life and your previous selfish behavior. These repercussions can be delayed for months, years, even lifetimes, according to Kabbalah.

The deception doesn't stop there. The Adversary has another trick up his sleeve.

REDIRECTING THE CONSEQUENCES

The Adversary can also redirect payback to another area of your life, further confusing you. In other words, if a person commits adultery, he or she is hurting his or her partner. This is not a sharing action. This is a receiving action. It creates distance and disconnection from the 99 Percent with darkness as the inevitable result. This darkness does not have to appear in a person's sex life. It may appear in business. It could manifest in relationship to a person's children. It can affect emotional well-being or even personal health. Because of the Adversary's use of redirection, we come to the mistaken conclusion that life is simply random, chaotic, based upon chance and luck.

We never connect the dots. We fail to realize that every selfish action (whether it's philandering or fighting with someone over a parking space) is subject to the law of *Cause and Effect*. Every negative action causes a negative reaction somewhere down the line.

THE PAYOFF

When we resist adultery, we generate tremendous amounts of Light in our life. This Light not only gets directed to our sexual relationships, but it also extends into areas of our life where we need it most. Remember, Light is the cure-all for everything that ails us. Our financial, emotional, and marital problems all stem from a lack of Light. Light delivers everything you need to be infinitely happy and fulfilled.

THE IMPORTANCE OF CONSCIOUSNESS

Consciousness and intent are key activators of kabbalistic technology. What does this mean? It means that if you choose to resist the temptation to cheat on your partner out of guilt, you will *not* arouse Light. Likewise, if you resist a little hanky panky out of fear of religious disapproval, it will also not work. Someone once asked me if God would punish him if he cheated on his wife. I told him bluntly: *God does not punish. God also does not reward.*

For instance, when a person sticks a finger in a wall plug socket, the force of electricity will shock him or her. It might even kill them. But did the force of electricity consciously punish them? Likewise, plug a lamp into that same force and you banish darkness from a room. The Force of God works the same way. How we connect to this powerful force determines whether you receive Light or pain. It's up to you.

SUPPRESSION IS MISSING THE POINT

We do not suppress feelings in Kabbalah. We do not resist certain behaviors out of fear or guilt. We do not give things up in Kabbalah. When we act from that consciousness, it means we don't understand how things really work. The truth of the matter is that students of Kabbalah are a greedy bunch. But we possess the ultimate form of greed—greed for the Light of the Creator. Too many people settle for the lowest form of greed there is—greed for the ego. The latter delivers only temporary pleasure. Ultimate greed delivers lasting fulfillment.

When you're faced with the temptation of a one-night stand, resist for the purpose of connecting to your 99 Percent Reality in order to get more happiness. Otherwise, what's the point?

THE BLESSING OF DIVORCE

Resistance is not a reason to remain imprisoned in a failed and unhappy marriage. The act of divorce is actually one of the precepts and blessings in Old Testament biblical law. If a marriage is destined to end, for whatever good reason, try to avoid outside sexual relationships until the divorce is finalized. Kabbalistically, the process of divorce safely disconnects the two souls from one another, so that no short circuits can take place during the breakup. Many times, two people enter into a marriage to work out karmic debts from a previous life; there are lessons to be learned and situations that must be experienced for growth purposes. However, once those debts are paid off, once those lessons are learned, a marriage can be dissolved so that both partners are free to evolve and move on to new relationships.

TOOLS TO RESIST CHEATING

The following passage of *Zohar* eradicates unwanted philandering impulses from our nature. Too late? Never. This powerful text also helps purify negative energy and darkness created as a result of infidelity. Everyone can get a clean start and begin to enrich their lives the moment they decide to do so.

MEDITATION

‎68. וְזִמְנִין קוּדְשָׁא בְּרִיךְ הוּא לְאַפָּקָא חַד רוּחָא דְּכָלִיל מִכֻּלְּהוּ. דִּכְתִּיב מֵאַרְבַּע רוּחוֹת בֹּאִי הָרוּחַ. אַרְבַּע רוּחוֹת בֹּאִי לָא כְּתִיב כָּאן, אֶלָּא מֵאַרְבַּע רוּחוֹת בֹּאִי. וּבְיוֹמֵי דְּמַלְכָּא מְשִׁיחָא, לָא יִצְטָרְכוּן לְמֵילַף חַד לְחַד, דְּהָא רוּחָא דִּלְהוֹן דְּכָלִיל מִכָּל רוּחִין. יָדְעַ בֹּלָּא. חָכְמָה וּבִינָה עֵצָה וּגְבוּרָה דַּעַת וְיִרְאַת יְיָ'. מִשּׁוּם רוּחָא דִּכְלִילָא מִכָּל רוּחֵי. בג״כ כְּתִיב, מֵאַרְבַּע רוּחוֹת, דְּאִינּוּן אַרְבַּע דִּכְלִילָן בְּשִׁבְעָה דַּרְגִּין עִלָּאִין דְּאַמְרָן. וְתָאנָא, דְּכֻלְּהוּ כְּלִילָן בְּהַאי רוּחָא דְּעַתִּיקָא דְּעַתִּיקִין, דְּנָפִיק מִמּוֹחָא סְתִימָאָה לְנוּקְבָא דְּחוֹטָמָא.

HOMOSEXUALITY

Kabbalah does not offer an opinion on this issue, quite simply because Kabbalah is not a religion or a philosophy with opinions about sexual orientation. Kabbalah is a blueprint, a technology based on the energy of life. It allows us to have more Light in our lives, to strengthen our connection to that 99 Percent Reality of spirituality from which we all derive.

Kabbalah explains that the ultimate purpose of life is to transform our selfish desires and learn to share with people. As we discussed earlier, relationships are the major part of this process. Everyone, gay or not, faces the tough task of learning to resist the overwhelmingly selfish behaviors the Adversary proposes. When any two people commit to taking that journey together, to being sharing and conscious of the effect their actions have on the world, they reveal great Light in the world.

When speaking with my gay students, I find that they easily connect to the idea of male and female energies. Remember, these are the positive and negative charges that exist in the unified soul. In fact, Kabbalah explains that male and female energies, or male and female souls, can be drawn into a body of the opposite sex. People can even have a combination of both these energies, which can affect their sexuality.

Ultimately, the soul of a person chooses the body it will inhabit before entering the physical world. And we are all here for the same reason: To learn to be more sharing, to become like the Light, and to ignite the Law of Attraction in our lives. So whatever combination of soul and body we may have, we are all exactly who we need to be in order to accomplish this mission. Kabbalah explains that wherever the fantastic voyage may take us, we are all sparks of the Divine, of the Creator, and the Creator does not make mistakes.

Treating all people with human dignity is an essential tool of Kabbalah. Not because it is morally correct, but because judgment and hatred are tools of our Adversary and they immediately disconnect us from the Light. Treating everyone with kindness, compassion, and sharing connects us to the Light that will infuse our own lives with passion and excitement.

> There are more things in heaven and Earth, Horatio, than are dreamt of in your philosophy.
> —William Shakespeare, *Hamlet*

It is important that we all understand the concept of male and female as they are defined kabbalistically. Male and female do not necessarily refer to a physical male and female body. Kabbalah deals with forces of energy that have nothing to do with materiality. There is male energy and female energy, and these two particular forces can be found in either a man's or a woman's physical body, in varying proportions. In gay relationships, it's not unusual to find that one partner expresses more female qualities and the other more male ones. This is a direct result of the particular male or female energy that shines in each person's soul.

Rachel is gay, and she has been a student of Kabbalah for three years. Before Kabbalah, Rachel was constantly filled with a fear of rejection. She had no idea what her purpose in life was, or how her sexuality fit into the scheme of things.

> Studying Kabbalah helped me realize that it isn't about whether you're gay or straight; it's about understanding that every single person has something to contribute to life. We're

all responsible for the amount of negativity or Light in the world. When you learn to resist the ego, it's like finding a new treasure every day. Instead of being bogged down by guilt and shame, boredom and emptiness, you're inspired to write the book you always dreamed of, volunteer to help abused kids like you've always meant to, or even just let go of grudges and pain you've carried around for years. It's not about what you want; it's about who you are.

A lot of times people focus on the sex part of homosexuality, which is understandable when you learn how much we all focus on the 1 percent of reality. But being gay is about a lot more than just sex. No one has a monopoly on being selfish in sex and relationships. We all do it. I realized that life is about making the effort to see that spark of the Creator in someone else and to really appreciate it. Especially in the people I disagree with the most, those who really push my buttons.

As a final thought on this subject, suppose we have a heterosexual couple that treats each other abusively. They mistreat their friends and business colleagues, and their behavior lacks any form of human decency.

Suppose we have a gay couple that shares a life distinguished by a constant striving to be kind toward others. They make an effort to treat people with human dignity. Which couple, according to the teachings of Kabbalah, reveals greater Light in the world?

Answer? (No surprise here.) The gay couple.

Allow me to paraphrase a teaching of the great kabbalistic sage known as Hillel:

> *The sole purpose of Bible study is to achieve the ability to love one's neighbor as oneself. All the rest of the learning is mere commentary. Now go and learn.*

ORGASMS: FEMALE FIRST

A famous medieval kabbalistic text called *The Book of the Pious* states the following:

> *Your wife should dress and adorn herself like a "fruitful vine"*
> *so that your lust will become inflamed like a fire, and you will*
> *shoot semen like an arrow . . . You should delay your orgasm*
> *until your wife has her orgasm first.*

Men usually reach orgasm first because they tend to be more easily aroused. However, a man should ensure that his wife experiences lots of pleasure during sex, and that she achieves orgasm first. According to Kabbalah, a man also has an obligation to satisfy his wife and give her sex on a regular basis. It is his responsibility, and not the other way around. If a man refuses to have sex with his wife when she requests it, it is actually grounds for divorce. Thus a women's pleasure and her orgasm are critically important in Kabbalah.

Let's find out why by examining the importance of foreplay.

THE SIGNIFICANCE OF KISSING, TOUCHING, AND FOREPLAY

Foreplay is a vital aspect of lovemaking, according to Kabbalah. Kissing, for example, is a powerful way to merge souls. Why? Breath is essentially an aspect of a person's soul. When breath is commingled through passionate kissing, the two souls unite.

Lovemaking without kissing and some serious foreplay is considered to be masturbation. And it cannot be simple little kisses. The kissing must be hot, passionate, and wild. Let's just say the French got it right when it comes to kissing Kabbalah style. As *The Zohar* states:

> *There are no kisses of joy and love **except** when they cling to each other, mouth-to-mouth, spirit-to-spirit, and saturate each other with pleasure and ecstasy.*

During foreplay, a male should devote all his energy to arousing his partner to the highest possible degree. Why? This leads us back to the very beginning of this book and the first Kabbalistic principle, which stated:

The Light of the Creator cannot manifest and express itself without a receiver.

When a woman is aroused, her sexual desire intensifies. She becomes a true and effective Receiver. She becomes a recipient for the Light to fill her from the Upper World.

The great medieval kabbalist Moses ben Nakhman wrote:

> *It is fitting to win her heart with words of charm and seduction and other proper things.*

The greater a woman's desire is, the more Light there is to fill her. This is a critically important concept. Kabbalah teaches that when a man and woman unite in passionate lovemaking, our 1 Percent World and the 99 Percent Reality *mirror this union*. This is not a metaphor. This is not an analogy. This is a fact.

This means that the stronger the desire of a woman, the more Light fills our 1 Percent World. The sexual arousal of a woman arouses all of physical existence and expands its ability to draw down the Light of the 99 Percent Reality. For this reason, the more a man seduces, arouses, and charms a woman—both prior to intercourse and during—the more Light the couple and our crazy, chaotic world will receive in turn.

WHY WOMEN FIRST

Believe it or not, lovemaking that embodies true sharing between a couple banishes darkness, pain, and suffering from the landscape of human existence. Only our Adversary prevents us from grasping the power of this truth. Likewise, selfish sex or abusive sex contributes only to more darkness to the world.

When a woman reaches orgasm first, her desire, her state-of-receiving is at its absolute peak. Now a man can impart his semen through his own orgasm, generating and sharing the maximum pleasure with his partner and with the world. If a man climaxes first, before a woman is fully aroused, she receives limited pleasure, if any at all. Her limited pleasure, in turn, reduces the amount of Light that is revealed in our world. If she gets nothing, the world gets nothing.

Let's examine this in a bit more detail.

THE MALE ORGASM

After or during a woman's orgasm, a man should ejaculate as quickly as he can, with as much intensity as possible. His ejaculation correlates to the Light filling the Soul. Moreover, at the precise moment a man ejaculates, his body is now in a pure and absolute state of sharing as he imparts this life force to his partner. Consequently, this seminal fluid discharge delivers the most exalted pleasure known to man.

In the midst of an orgasm, the Light of the Creator is permeating a man's entire being as it flows through him for those few mystical moments. A man has now attained a state of oneness with the Light of the Creator via the Law of Attraction, for both he and the Light now have identical sharing natures.

However, ejaculation is an automatic mode of sharing. Once a climax is achieved, there is no Free Choice as the semen shoots out automatically. Thus, a man's state of oneness and his intense pleasure are heavenly but brief. The precise moment the male's auto-state of sharing (ejaculation) ends, the pleasure ceases, and he returns to this physical existence.

SHARING AND THE JOY OF AN ORGASM

Kabbalists tell us that an orgasm gives us a tiny taste of what it truly feels like to behave like God. In other words, genuine sharing is actually an orgasmic experience. We feel it during sex. But, unfortunately, sharing in other parts of our life feels like the exact opposite of an orgasm. It's uncomfortable. We hate sharing. We do not like giving something away. We don't like giving till it hurts—precisely because it *does hurt!* We love receiving. We love getting.

These opposite feelings arise by design. The true orgasmic joy of sharing is purposely concealed from our senses so that we may exercise legitimate free will when we choose to resist receiving and, instead, share with others. This makes perfect sense when you stop and think about it. Just imagine if every time you did a sharing action you felt the joy of an incredible orgasm.

> You give money to a worthy charitable cause . . . *Orgasm!*
> You contribute time to help the elderly . . . *Orgasm!*
> You assist your spouse with household chores . . . *Orgasm!*
> You feed the hungry . . . *Orgasm!*
> You volunteer and help build housing for the homeless . . . *Orgasm!*
> You offer your competitor in business genuine help . . . *Orgasm!*
> You offer your worst enemy kindness and love . . . *Orgasm!*

If simple acts of sharing produced mind-blowing orgasms each and every time, you can bet your bottom dollar that the entire world would be hysterically running around trying to share with as many people as possible.

Ironically, people everywhere are already running around day and night trying to achieve an orgasm. Everything they do, in truth, contains a hidden agenda that eventually leads to the goal of having great sex. But they are doing it by way of receiving, and not by sharing. Because most of us have things backwards, the world is engulfed by greed, and therefore by darkness and chaos.

Now imagine this: What if the orgasm you experienced from sharing was actually 60 times more powerful than the one you had last week? Yes, this planet would become one big orgy of generosity! Sharing, kindness, brotherhood, sisterhood, goodwill, and positive deeds would break out all over the world, spreading faster than the world's most infectious virus.

OUR FINAL DESTINY

It just so happens that this is precisely what's in store for all of us once we remove the Adversary from our nature and from this world once and for all. After we complete the job of resisting 100 percent, the last curtain will be pulled back, and the joy associated with true sharing will be revealed and experienced by all humanity.

You will be seeking out sharing opportunities to help fill the needs of your fellow man because of the orgasmic joy it brings you. What's even more incredible is that six billion other souls will be busying themselves 24 hours a day trying to share all of their good fortune with you. Everyone will be busy feeding and caring for their fellow men and women, copping an orgasm in the process. You will be sharing. And you will be receiving gifts from billions of other people. Whew! What a scenario!

Naturally, it's difficult to believe all of this because the Adversary is still among us. Your doubts and skepticism are his doing.

Thankfully, we have the tools of Kabbalah to help us pierce this illusion and banish these doubts so that we may all achieve ultimate fulfillment sooner rather than later.

By the way, the ultimate reward of this transformation of human behavior goes far beyond the pleasure of an orgasm. Let's discover the ultimate payoff by examining one more kind of orgasm. A woman's.

THE FEMALE ORGASM

When a woman achieves orgasm during intercourse, she is actually in a state of *Receiving for the Sake of Sharing*. In other words, she is receiving the male sex organ and, by doing so, she is imparting pleasure to her partner. It is important for a woman to be aware of this. She must maintain a conscious intent to receive pleasure for the purpose of sharing pleasure with her partner. If a woman is thinking only about herself, her receiving becomes just an act of receiving. This disconnects her from the 99 Percent.

But if she realizes that she is imparting love and pleasure to her partner, her act of receiving, according to Kabbalah, is suddenly transformed into an act of sharing. This idea is deep and profoundly important.

When a woman alters her consciousness so that she is receiving sexual pleasure, including her orgasm, for the sole purpose of imparting pleasure to her partner, she is now in a pure state of sharing. As a result, she joins her soul to the 99 Percent, and she receives tremendous pleasure as well. This, by the way, is the ultimate paradox. The more a man and woman think only about sharing, the more they receive in return. What's more, a woman's sharing consciousness charges the sexual battery in her relationship, ensuring continued passionate intimate relations in the future.

A MICROCOSM OF CREATION

A man and woman in the throes of an orgasm are in the exact same relationship as the Light and Soul in the original Creation. Sex with the right consciousness embodies the ultimate goal of Creation:

The Light Sharing with the Soul
The Soul Receiving Pleasure for the Sake of Sharing with the Creator

In this dynamic, both the Light and Soul are considered to be sharing.

Remember the Garden of Eden? Do you recall what the Serpent told the Soul during their fateful game? The Serpent said that if the Soul could receive for the sole purpose of sharing with the Creator, the receiving trait of the Soul would suddenly transform into a sharing trait. Thus, both the Light and Soul would be in a state of sharing. The whole purpose of life on Earth is to transform our selfish *Desire to Receive* into a *Desire to Receive for the Sake of Sharing*.

Sexual intercourse represents the most powerful and meaningful way to achieve this dynamic.

If a man thinks about his wife first, and focuses on sharing with her instead of his own orgasm, he is a perfect model of the Light: unconditional sharing.

If a woman considers her husband first, receiving all the pleasure that he is giving her for the sole purpose of imparting pleasure to him, she is now a perfect model of the Soul. She is Receiving for the Sake of Sharing. Her receiving is now considered to be an act of sharing. After all, nothing makes a man happier than seeing his partner overwhelmed with desire and pleasure as a result of his magnificent lovemaking.

Both the male and female are now in a pure state of sharing. Get the idea? They can now achieve oneness together because of their identical natures. What's more, they now attain oneness and connection with the Light of the Creator. Not only that, but in that one blissful moment, the *entire* cosmos mirrors their sexual union. Our world has intercourse with the 99 Percent Reality.

This is how we transform our world and transform our personal sex lives. It's about giving, not receiving. It's about using our desires in a positive sharing manner.

The benefits don't end with great sex and world transformation. We're also talking about the secret for achieving immortality. Immortality is the ultimate payoff once we master the art of *Receiving for the Sake of Sharing*.

SEX AND IMMORTALITY

If you want to discover a few ancient kabbalistic secrets about achieving genuine immortality, keep reading. If you want to jump ahead to some more sex tips, skip this next section.

Do you know why people die? Not because of disease. Not because of old age. Not because of illness. That's just the effect. It's not the cause. People die because their atoms stop holding hands. Allow me to explain.

Everything in the world is made up of atoms. Everything!

Footballs. Fettuccini. Fonzi. Molecules. Ballistic missiles. Steamed mussels. Pebbles on the beach. Clouds in the sky. Stars in the heavens. Incan idols in ancient Peruvian temples. American Idols currently on Fox TV.

There is nothing in our universe that is not made up of atoms. So why is there so much diversity in the world? Why does a heart look different from a kidney if both are made up of atoms? For the same reason that *words* can have vastly different meanings even though they're composed of the exact same letters of the alphabet. It all depends how the letters or atoms are arranged.

THE BUILDING BLOCKS OF LIFE

Consider Lego building blocks. You can build a car, a rocket, a robot, a building, or practically anything else with Lego. It all depends how you arrange the blocks. Likewise, atoms arranged in one way create brain tissue. Atoms arranged another way create the *National Enquirer*. Clearly, these are dissimilar forms of matter (in more ways than one).

I WANNA HOLD YOUR HAND

Atoms group together by creating bonds with one another. In simpler terms, they *hold hands*. When two or more atoms *hold hands*, they are now called molecules. Molecules are simply a bunch of atoms holding hands together. Molecules then form together to create all physical matter, from alligators to zucchini.

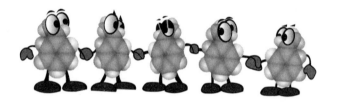

ATOMS BONDED TOGETHER CREATE A MOLECULE.

WHEN THE BOND BREAKS

When atoms stop holding hands, they break apart. That's when a molecule ceases to exist. We see this as deterioration.

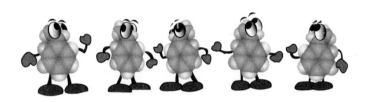

**BONDS BETWEEN ATOMS BREAK,
CREATING INDIVIDUAL ATOMS. THE MOLECULE NO LONGER EXISTS.**

THE INDESTRUCTIBLE ATOM

Science has shown us, irrefutably, that atoms themselves never die or wear out. Atoms are indestructible. So when atoms stop holding hands, the molecule might die, but the individual atoms that made up the molecule live forever. The atoms that support your existence are billions of years old.

Once again, consider Lego. Suppose you build a man out of Lego building blocks. When you take apart all the Lego pieces, the man dies. But the individual Lego pieces live on.

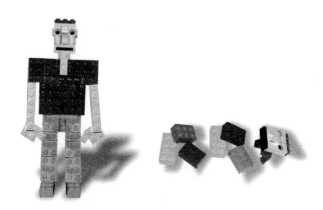

Likewise, when a human being dies, the individual atoms that built that man live on. In fact, physics tells us that these atoms are as brand spanking new as they were the day that person was born. The person's atoms simply circulate back into the Earth and atmosphere.

So the ultimate question is this: Why do the atoms that make up our body stop holding hands? If they didn't, wouldn't we achieve immortality? That's absolutely correct.

Most scientists never even consider the big picture. They deal with the symptoms of diseases that occur as a result of atoms no longer holding hands, but they don't ask the question: *Why makes atoms stop holding hands?*

Kabbalah asks this ultimate question.
Kabbalah also answers it.

When Kabbalah revealed the answer to this question 2,000 years ago, it was called mysticism. Why? Because the atom had not yet been discovered. Consequently, the lay person had no idea what the kabbalists were referring to when they spoke about the various positive and negative forces that are found inside an atom. As we saw earlier, atoms are made up of

- protons,

- electrons,

- neutrons.

We also discovered:

- The proton is really the Light and the force of Sharing (+).

- The electron is really the Soul and the force of Receiving (-).

- The neutron is the concept of Resistance.

The key here is the electron, or the *Desire to Receive*, which are one and the same force.

WHAT THE ATOM REALLY IS

At its most profound level, an atom is actually consciousness. That's it. That's all that really exists, anyway. When we travel back to the moment of Creation, we can see the force underlying all matter for what it really is.

- There is the consciousness of the Light, the positive force of Sharing.

- There is the consciousness of the Soul, the negative force of Receiving.

- And there is the consciousness of the Soul's act of Resistance, which is what brought about the Creation of our world in the first place.

These three forms of consciousness are what create an atom. It's that simple.

HOW ATOMS HOLD HANDS

Atoms hold hands by virtue of the electron. In scientific terms, *atoms share electrons* and this is how they bond together. When atoms no longer share their electrons, it means they are no longer holding hands. Slowly, our Lego man is being disassembled. When enough atoms stop holding hands, death occurs.

The fact that the electron is the key player when it comes to atoms holding hands is, kabbalistically, elegant and stunning. The electron is being utilized in a sharing fashion. Get it? We came here to transform our *Desire to Receive* (the electron) into a *Desire to Receive for the Sake of Sharing* (atoms sharing electrons).

Think about the profundity of all of this. And do not let the language and the terminology confuse you.

The kabbalistic phrase:

Desire to Receive for the Sake of Sharing

Is the exact same idea as:

Electrons Being Shared by Atoms

The only reason atoms stop holding hands is that our consciousness is stuck in a *Desire to Receive for the Self Alone*. This is the Adversary. And this is the ultimate cause of death. And this is why The Bible says the Serpent brought death to this world. Death is caused by selfishness and the concept of non-stop receiving without any aspect of sharing.

Every time we react selfishly, every time we receive and refuse to share, a few hundred atoms or so stop holding hands. A few more molecules cease to exist. This shows up as aging, wear and tear on the body, illness, disease, and every other form of chaos and decay.

When we resist and remove the Adversary from our consciousness forever, once and for all, we will be in a perfect state of *Receiving for the Sake of Sharing*. In other words, the atoms (which are nothing but a reflection of our consciousness) will forever share the electron and thus, never stop holding hands. Atoms are immortal. If they hold hands forever, our bodies become immortal, and we live forever.

This is a simple explanation of how immortality will be achieved in our world. This is also the secret meaning behind Kabbalah's essential teaching:

Love Thy Neighbor as Thyself.

Loving yourself is Receiving.

Loving your Neighbor is Sharing.

Loving your Neighbor as You Love Yourself is simply another way of saying: *Receiving (Love) for the Sake of Sharing (Love).*

This is why it's known as the Golden Rule. It's the path to immortality. Moses knew this. Jesus knew this. The prophet Muhammad knew this. The reason the Torah, The New Testament and The Koran speak about destroying one's enemy is that the *enemy within* must be wiped out! The enemy is a code word for the Adversary. Unfortunately, it has taken religion thousands of years to realize the true meaning of the word *enemy*.

The Adversary is all about Receiving Selfishly. When we destroy this enemy and we *Receive for the Sake of Sharing*, immortality will be ours for the taking. This is why Moses, Jesus, and Muhammad declared that eternal life would be achieved at the End of Days. The End of Days means the End of the Adversary. But it's up to us to make it happen.

SEX AS A MEANS TO IMMORTALITY

We can now begin to perceive the significance of sex. Sex is the perfect opportunity to build the ultimate model of *Sharing* and *Receiving for the Sake of Sharing*.

When we achieve this dynamic, our sex life lives forever!

Likewise, when we hold hands with our partner, when we hold hands with all the people in our lives, sharing friendship and offering love unconditionally, the atoms in our bodies will hold hands with each other unconditionally.

Immortality will become the new reality.

RESISTING SEX DURING THE MEN-STRUAL CYCLE

During a woman's menstrual cycle, there is no resistance taking place between the blood (red, negative charge) and the sperm (white, positive energy). In other words, if sexual relations occur, the positive force (+) connects directly to the negative charge (-) causing a short circuit. This produces a huge power drain. Actually, consider it a meltdown.

In addition, when this blood is expelled from a woman, this is considered to be a broken vessel, a shattering of a soul, which was once ready to give life. This shattering correlates to the shattering of the One Soul in our Creation story. Thus, we do not want to connect to this energy.

When a couple makes love with the intent to have a child, and the egg is fertilized by the sperm, the menstrual cycle stops and the woman connects to an energy of Light and sharing. Milk, for example, is created within her body, which will eventually sustain the newborn infant. This transformation in the Soul, of red blood into white milk, occurs only when sperm fertilizes the egg—when Light fills the Soul. A sharing cycle occurs when conception takes place.

We have

- male sharing with female,

- female sharing with male,

- sperm sharing with egg, and

- mother sharing with child.

During menstruation, there is no potential for this sharing cycle. There is no soul to hold the Light of creation and human life. For that reason, we do not connect white sperm with red blood. Resisting sex during this period flips on the Light.

THE TECHNIQUE

According to Kabbalah, it is best to abstain from sex during a woman's monthly flow from the first sign of blood and for seven days from the time she is free of spotting, usually a twelve-day time frame.

For our male readers who find the prospect of going twelve days without an orgasm too challenging, consider this: Be happy you're human. Penguins reach orgasm only once a year. Besides, there is an upside.

The seven additional days of abstinence, from the time a woman's period is over correlates to the Seven Dimensions in the 99 Percent Realm and Seventh Heaven. The Light from Seventh Heaven flows down through seven dimensions into the woman's soul. During this seven-day period, a woman's soul is rebuilt, and she is born anew. And that's a good thing, because the relationship between husband and wife is born anew during this stage. Sex after this time lapse feels like *sex for the first time!* Passions soar!

After this time has passed, on the night when sex will be taking place, a woman can also immerse herself in water thirteen times. Dipping in the ocean, a pool, or an actual ritual bath is a powerful way to conclude the menstrual phase and prepare a woman's soul to be a powerful recipient and vessel for the Light of the Creator.

Remember Michael and Meredith? They began using this kabbalistic tool and found that it resurrected their sex lives in ways they never imagined.

MICHAEL:
Before Kabbalah, we could go months without having sex. When we finally did it, it was still boring. All that down time did nothing to generate excitement. When we tried not having sex during my wife's period after studying Kabbalah, the first night was unbelievable. There was this nervous sexual tension that made me feel like I was eighteen. It wasn't just about being apart for a period of time. Something internal was happening. Everything felt new.

When we first tried this technique, it was difficult as hell. We failed a few times. I was like a caged tiger. I was in a rotten mood. We fought a lot during those seven days. I was a real asshole. But we continued trying. After a few months I finally got used to it. I was shocked at how incredible it was on that first night of sex. That's what always gave me the motivation to get through those twelve days. I was like a teenager, dreaming and fantasizing about having sex with my wife all day long. When that night finally arrives, we literally tear our clothes off.

MEREDITH:
Sex with my husband was boring. For me it was a waste of time. I did it to keep the peace between us. I no longer had any desire. I remember the first time we kept the twelve days. On the night we had sex, it was totally wild for me! Every month was the same. The anticipation was intense. I never believed that sex could be like they show in films. Now I feel like I am

having the kind of sex you see in movies. But there was some-thing more important. I noticed that my husband began respecting me more. He became more sensitive. He was more considerate toward me. That was an unexpected surprise. In fact, that was more important to me than the great sex. He became a more gentle and loving person. He was no longer a jerk.

ADDITIONAL SUGGESTIONS FOR GREAT SEX

SEXUAL POSITIONS

Remember the old black-and-white TV sets with rabbit-ear antennae? How you moved the antenna—the way it was positioned—determined the strength and quality of the signal. Our bodies work the same way. The position of the body during sex determines the quality and strength of sexual signal and the Light it receives. Kabbalists have revealed various techniques to draw the highest frequency of Light and the strongest signal.

MISSIONARY

Great position. Highly recommended, especially during the moment of orgasm. Why? A male correlates to the Upper World. A female embodies our Lower World. Thus, a man on top emulates the position of the spiritual worlds. There is perfect alignment between man and woman and the Upper and Lower Worlds. This ensures the maximum flow of Light into our lives and into this physical existence during orgasm.

WOMAN ON TOP

This works well during the initial stages of intercourse. But at the moment of orgasm, if the couple rolls over and consummates their lovemaking in the missionary position, you generate a more powerful connection to Light. Most important, if your consciousness is tuned into the reason why—aligning yourselves with the Upper and Lower Worlds—the intensity of the orgasm will be even greater.

MAN BEHIND WITH THE WOMAN ON ALL FOURS

The pleasure we feel from this position originates from the lowest grade of soul in our being, our animal instinct.

This position, a favorite with many people, is reserved for the animal kingdom. Our unique purpose in this world, however, is to elevate to a higher level of existence. Thus, when we forego this position—*with the intent to connect to spiritual Light and elevate our souls*—the pleasure generated from the missionary position will be *far greater* than any pleasure you have previously experienced from this rear position.

In other words, if we cannot feel and experience the benefit, why do it? Kabbalists would not prescribe or discourage a practice unless there was a greater benefit to be received.

If you still feel inclined to use this position, perhaps use it for arousal purposes and return to the missionary position during the moment of orgasm.

ORAL SEX

Kabbalah recommends using oral sex for arousal purposes. However, a man should not ejaculate this way, for this leaves the semen exposed. When semen is exposed, negative forces immediately attach themselves to it and rob us of our Light. When a couple consummates their oral foreplay with sexual intercourse, greater Light is injected into their relationship.

SEX UNDER THE INFLUENCE

If one or both partners are under the influence of drugs or alcohol, the Light that is generated goes to the Adversary. The couple's sexual battery is drained.

Sex under the influence also includes being under the influence of anger or hostility. If there is anger or hatred in our hearts toward our partner, and we engage in sex merely to experience personal pleasure, this is considered a major short circuit. Once again, the Light goes to our Adversary. We are left holding a bag of negative energy that will cause chaos in our life.

Keep in mind there is no problem having a drink together to relax and unwind. But drinking a few bottles to induce a drunken state inevitably backfires.

RESIST PREMARITAL SEX

A soul mate connection means two halves of one soul have at last found one another after many lifetimes. They are now ready to be merged into one. But what is the glue that allows these two opposite forms to unite? It is the marriage vow. Once again, we can turn to the metaphor of a light bulb to see how sexual energy is created in a marriage.

A light bulb has a positive pole (+) and a negative pole (-). These are opposite forces that somehow must come together to create a working relationship. If they connect directly, they short-circuit. The bulb burns out. The relationship between the two opposite forces is kaput! The key to uniting these opposite forms is the filament. The filament creates resistance, which unites the positive and negative so that, together, they work to generate light.

A man corresponds to the *positive pole* in a bulb.

A woman corresponds to the *negative pole* in a bulb.

The wedding vows and the institution of marriage is the *filament* that bonds and unites these two opposite forces, thus allowing the two halves of one soul to work together and create spiritual Light.

Sex before marriage is simply a direct connection and short circuit, lacking a filament. If we resist the desire for premarital sex (the filament), and we wait until we have incorporated the oath of marriage into the relationship, we arouse enduring Light.

This is about smart and shrewd investing in spiritual assets. When we abstain with intent to create a circuit of energy between oneself and the Light, sexual energy is stored away and continues to grow as you keep investing more Light for the long term.

TOOLS FOR RESISTANCE

For those who would like try this practice, there are passages of *The Zohar* that help us control our sexual desires.

Visually scan and/or meditate upon *The Zohar* verse below. Each word, each letter radiates a spiritual force that releases sexual tension, while, at the same time, building up and preserving your sexual energy for a lifetime of sexual bliss with your spouse.

MEDITATION

328. ר' אַבָּא אֲמַר, מַאי דִכְתִיב וְאֶת שַׁבְּתוֹתַי קַדֵּשׁוּ, אֶלָּא אֵין עוֹנָתָן שֶׁל תָּא חֲזֵי, אֶלָּא מִשַּׁבָּת לְשַׁבָּת, וּמַזְהַר לְהוֹ, דְּהוֹאִיל דְּתַשְׁמִישׁ הַמִּטָּה דְּמִצְוָה הוּא, קַדֵּשׁוּ. כְּלוֹמַר, קַדְשׁוּ עַצְמְכֶם בְּשַׁבְּתוֹתַי, בְּהַהוּא תַּשְׁמִישׁ דְּמִצְוָה אָמַר רַב יְהוּדָה אָמַר רַב, הַאי מַאן דְּעָיֵיל לְקַרְתָּא, וְחָמֵי נַשֵׁי שַׁפִּירָן יַרְכִּין עֵינוֹי, וְיֵימָא הָכִי סָךְ סְפָאן, אִיגְזַר אִיגְזַרְנָא קָרְדִינָא תְּקִיל פּוֹק פּוֹק, דַּאֲבוֹי קַדִּישָׁא דְּשַׁבַּתָּא הוּא. מ"ט דַּחֲמִימוּת דְּאָרְחָא שָׁלַט בֵּיהּ, וְיָכִיל יצה"ר לְשַׁלְטָא עֲלוֹי.

FRIDAY NIGHT SEX

I'm gonna wait 'til the midnight hour . . . that's when my love comes tumbling down.
    —Wilson Picket

Kabbalah tells us that sexual connections on Friday night, especially after midnight, are greatly enhanced by cosmic energy forces that are available during this unique period. Here's what happens: Every Friday evening, at the stroke of midnight, our entire 1 Percent Reality elevates and draws near to the 99 Percent Reality. A window opens up. The curtain is pulled back. If you now pull back the sheets and climb into bed, an ocean of spiritual energy awaits you. Two people coming together on Friday night will cause the physical world to come together with the spiritual world In the closest connection possible. The result is divine sex. The result is a world bathed in sacred Light.

ROLLING NAKED IN THE SNOW

Sure, it sounds bizarre, but the revered Renaissance Kabbalist Rav Isaac Luria recommended rolling in the snow, naked, to purify and remove any and all negative blockages that have been created as a result of 1 Percent Selfish Sex. These blockages prevent sexual energy from flowing into our lives.

Remember, the Light is always there. If you have a room with a lamp burning brightly and you cover that lamp with twenty-two layers of curtain, the room is pitch black. But the light is still shining. The problem is the curtain. Each time you remove a layer of curtain, the room gets a bit brighter. Each of these tools pulls back the curtains in our lives. Rolling in the snow stark naked just happens to remove a heck of a lot of curtains at one time.

Water, according to kabbalah, is one of the closest substances on Earth to the Light of the Creator. Science tells us that H_2O is one of the most mysterious elements in the universe. For this reason, water is used for both physical and spiritual purification purposes.

Water, in the form of snow, is a powerful cleansing tool. It removes lifetimes of selfish sexual short circuits that have created more curtains than a dozen drapery manufacturers.

Jack is a student of Kabbalah who experienced rolling naked in the snow. Here is his story:

SNOW WHITE ADVENTURE
At first, I absolutely refused to do it. I thought the whole idea

was insane. After a few months, however, I thought it might be a cool experience. After all, if the ancient kabbalists were getting together in the middle of the night 500 years ago to roll in the snow, it might be worth trying. It sort of reminded me of the polar bear club where people jump into a freezing lake in the middle of the winter as an annual ritual. Anyway, it was March in Los Angeles. Naturally, there was no snow on the ground. So five of us—three guys and two girls—piled into a Land Cruiser, and we headed up into the mountains. We left for the mountains late in the evening to arrive around midnight. We drove up the mountain, and the road became increasingly narrow as we climbed. Then the snow started appearing. And the temperature dropped fast. We went from 60 degrees at the bottom of the mountain to 12 degrees fifteen minutes later. It was scary driving up the mountain because it was totally dark. The road was covered in snow and ice. The elevation was around 6,000 feet.

We finally pulled over and stopped. It was so dark you could not see what was out there beyond the edge of the road. The girls closed their eyes and the guys got undressed. Then the guys closed their eyes and the girls followed the same routine and left to find their own area away from the guys in which to roll in the snow. I made sure the car was running in case of an emergency and, of course, to keep the heat on. I have to tell you, it's a bizarre feeling sitting naked in your car at the top of a mountain in the middle of the night and the temperature outside is only twelve degrees. It took a lot of courage to open that car door and step outside. But I did it. We started walking toward the trees. My feet sank into the snow. Suddenly, I could no longer feel them at all! They were totally numb. It's the same numbness you get when a dentist freezes your mouth. I felt like I was walking on two stubs. It freaked me out. We found a spot to roll in. I remember looking up and being amazed by the all the stars. It was a magnificent sight. You just don't see that kind of stunning, star-studded sky in the city.

Anyway, we were supposed to do nine complete rolls. I got down in the snow and started to roll, meditating to cleanse and purify my body and soul. After the first three rolls, the snow burned and cut. I almost chickened out from doing the rest. But then I just gathered my strength and finished. The snow was kind of hard and I got cut up pretty bad on my legs and butt. When it was over I was as high as a kite. The feeling was indescribable. That night I had the most amazing dreams. It's hard to describe, but let's just say that the power and truth of this tool became clear to me that night, and even more important, in my sexual relationship.

Below are instructions along with ancient kabbalistic meditations that we should scan before we roll. Bring along a towel and a warm blanket.

INSTRUCTIONS FOR ROLLING IN THE SNOW

Meditate upon the following kabbalistic passage from the writings of the great 16th century Kabbalist, Rav Isaac Luria, before rolling in the snow. Then roll nine times, starting and ending face down. The most effective way to roll is in units of three:

1. Lie face down in the snow and roll three times and then stand up.

2. Repeat the above exercise two more times (and then grab your towel)!

As this experience is unique for each individual, it is suggested that you get the advice of a Kabbalah teacher or a Student Support Instructor at 1-800-KABBALAH if you would like more details.

מי שמתגלגל ט' גלגולים, יכוין ליחד ולחבר ט' אותיות של ג' הי"ה דג' אהי"ה הנז', שהם סוד ו"ת של ג' פרצופים הנזכר, עם אלפין שבעולע ראשונות שלהם, הרי ט'.

UNITING THE
1 PERCENT AND
99 PERCENT

The following are ancient kabbalistic Aramaic letters that directly correspond to the Upper World and the Lower World. When we meditate upon these two symbols during the precise moment of orgasm, we unite the two realms. This helps to intensify the pleasure and increase the volume of Light that flows into our relationship and the physical world.

It restores the Light that was lost in the Garden of Eden. And it helps repair the original shattered One Soul, bringing our world closer to its ultimate destiny of peace and paradise.

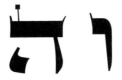

LOWER WORD   UPPER WORLD

Also, if you are trying to conceive a child, this meditation draws down the most positive and elevated souls from the Upper World. If you are not trying to conceive a child, your meditation *still* draws down elevated souls but directs them to other couples who are trying to conceive.

Since it's unlikely that you will bring this book into your bed so that you can meditate during the peak of your passion, try to memorize these images so that you can recall them when you need to. It may take you a few times. Or, you can meditate on them before sex.

RESIST SHAME
AND GUILT

Shame is a worthless, destructive, smothering emotion. It holds us back from being the loving, sharing people we were meant to be. It keeps us from having a true understanding of our desires, and it blocks the pathway to communicating with our spiritual aspect. That's why banishing shame is the first step to achieving a better sex life.

Shame is a deep-seated feeling that there is something wrong with you because of who you are, what you do, what you believe, or what may have happened to you in life. People can feel sexual shame if they are convinced that their sexual needs or desires are somehow dirty, embarrassing, or disgraceful. Nothing could be far-ther from the truth.

No matter where you came from, how you were raised, what you did in the past, or what you've believed until now, you need to know that sex is natural and beautiful. Sex, with the right intention, is how people connect with each other and connect with God. How could there be anything shameful in that?

Sex, done wrong, can be corrected and transformed through sex done right. Shame often blocks us from righting our wrongs. It's a trap. Forget about shame. Let it go.

SEXUAL ABUSE

Sadly, too many people were abused as children. Many more are abused as adults. One in every four girls is abused before the age of eighteen; one in every six boys is abused. The effects of sexual abuse are like scar tissue that continues to affect and influence behavior in various ways. These scars can lead to drug and alcohol abuse, low self-worth, divorce, distrust, lack of intimacy, shame, feelings of guilt, and self-destructive patterns in life and in relationships.

Please remember the following: Negative feelings, shameful emotions, guilt and worry are all connected to the 1 Percent Illusion, your Adversary. As difficult as it might be, you need to understand that someone might abuse your body, but in truth they can never abuse your soul, the authentic You.

No matter how deeply your guilt, pain, and shame penetrate, they never reach to your soul, which remains a perfect spark of the divine.

All of us have many, many layers of 1 Percent emotional suffering within us. But these layers, as painful as they are, never reach the soul. As we've seen, if we place a cloth over a lantern, the light dims, and each new layer of cloth further dims the light. But, in truth, the source of light never changes. The lantern remains constant. The lantern is unchanged. Your soul works the same way. It is shining brightly right now, as brightly as it did when it was first created by the Force we call God. The pains we feel in life are the blockages, the layers of cloth that have been placed over our soul.

Unfortunately, these blockages run deep. When abuse occurs, another cloth is placed over our essence. This dims the Light that comes from our soul, but the soul's original Light is always shining in full splendor.

When you share with others, when you make the attempt to resist guilt for the purpose of connecting to the 99 Percent, when you meditate upon *The Zohar*, when you learn all of these kabalistic truths, you gradually lift the layers of cloth that have dimmed your true self.

Know in your heart of hearts that all your pain can be healed.

WHAT'S SO GREAT ABOUT SHARING?

By now, you are probably beginning to see that all these tools and the entire body of wisdom known as Kabbalah are really just techniques for mastering the art of Sharing. At first, the whole idea of Sharing seems like a frightening proposition. We think Sharing means that somehow in some way we are going to wind up with less. And who in their right mind wants to wind up with less? But that whole notion is just a deception.

When you Share, you unite with God. You become God. And when you are God, you can create anything. That's the payoff. That's the reward for Sharing. Sharing is not about morals. Sharing is not about ethical behavior. It's about greed! Greed for the soul.

If you cut away a piece of a mountain, you now have a rock. The rock is no longer called a mountain only because it has been separated from its source. If you carefully place the rock back into the mountain, the rock and mountain suddenly become indistinguishable. The rock becomes the mountain.

When we are separated from God, we are called humans. And that means we are stuck with our human nature and our faulty, limited human traits. We are stuck with our chaos and are mired in turmoil. What causes our separation? Selfishness! Selfishness is just another term for the concept of receiving for the ego.

So every time we engage in behavior that feeds our ego, any time we react to anything, we are cut off from the Light. Instead of lasting pleasure and joy, we receive a temporary, momentary spark of pleasure. Instead of being Divine, we become mortal and flawed.

Receiving is the singular trait that created distance between us and the Light in the first place. When, however, you share, truly share until it hurts, then you unite with God (The Law of Attraction), and you become God. Now you can achieve anything and receive everything.

Of course, this is easier said than done. It's one thing to grasp the idea and a far different thing to internalize, practice, and live it in a self-indulgent world where you're told you have to step on other people in order to get ahead.

So the kabbalists gave us the tools we need to diminish the ego and stop the dead-end cycle of receiving and reactive behavior. This is how we find true love and achieve great sex! By the way, Kabbalah views love a whole lot differently than we might expect.

LOVE OR NEED?

Probably 99 percent of all people seek a loving relationship because they crave the warm feeling and sense of security that being loved provides. If you ask people why they love their partners, they usually say something like . . .

> He/she treats me with kindness.
> He/she makes me feel loved and appreciated.
> He/she is my best friend.
> I can confide in him/her.
> He/she really knows and understands me.
> He/she fulfills all my needs.
> He/she makes me feel safe, secure and happy.

From the kabbalistic perspective, there is something drastically wrong with that picture. According to kabbalists, that is not love. That is need! It's all about me. *It's all about what I am receiving, not what I am giving.*

Need is a self-centered desire. Need is a reactive trait. It eventually separates you from the Light, because the Law of Attraction says opposite forces repel one another. This is why most relationships fail. Instead of sharing, people are receiving.

UNCONDITIONAL IS THE KEY

Genuine love is about unconditional Sharing with another soul. The key word here is *unconditional*. The world uses that word a lot but few of us really get it or live it. Unconditional means there is no agenda.

There are no strings attached to the love one gives. There is no consideration given to what one will receive in return.

True love means a person finds joy is in the act of giving and seeing the happiness and fulfillment of the other person. That is love!

But that kind of love can evolve only through Resistance. The truth of the matter is we are constantly bombarded with self-centered desires. That's how the human body works. That's how the game of life operates. When, however, you Resist self-centered desires, and put the interests of your partner ahead of your own, you connect to Light. Guess what? That infusion of Light makes you a more loving and caring person. It also makes you happier in the end.

As you continue to Resist reactive, selfish behavior, your soul begins to grow and expand measure for measure. Slowly you learn how to love and share unconditionally. It's a process. It's a transformation. And it can take a lifetime to fully perfect your soul. But along the way, with each and every step, you can enjoy passionate and wild sex with your partner simply by utilizing this wisdom and the tools it provides.

YOUR INDIVIDUALITY: A FINAL WORD ABOUT THE LAW OF ATTRACTION

The Law of Attraction tells us that similarity creates closeness, and dissimilarity creates distance. Does this mean that soul mates must possess identical attributes and opinions about life? Are relationships and great sex really about two people being carbon copies of one another? Must we forsake our individuality and merely become identical to the other person?

No. Not in the least.

For instance, the similarity between two people can be seen in the area of spiritual goals, personal ideals, and human principles, but each person can still retain opposing opinions about such things as favorite movies and solutions to a problem. Consider a business with two partners. There is one singular goal shared by both partners: increased profits and expansion. The two partners are identical in this desire. They have the same goal, the same product, and they share identical business objectives. However, one partner is a financial wizard, and the other is marketing genius. Here we have two opposite roles serving one common goal. One partner uses the left brain. The other uses the right brain. These are opposite roles and traits. The marketing genius wants to spend, spend, spend in order to drive sales and thus increase profit. The financial wizard wants to curb all spending and costs in order to increase profits. Both are right. Sometimes the gung-ho marketing strategy is appropriate. Sometimes the frugal financial approach works best. The back and forth between the two partners and the business climate of the times all help to determine the right balance to grow the business and increase the bottom line.

If both partners treat each other proactively, with dignity, respect and unconditional love by using the technique of Resistance, a synergy is created between opposites and they unite. Remember, they are already close on one level because of their identical business and financial objectives. In the areas where they are opposed, they unite through the power of Resistance.

This is also the key to electrifying sex and the key to passionate, loving, and successful relationships. Two individuals merge together, completing one another. They are two halves of a single soul. They have repaired one aspect of the shattered soul by becoming true soul mates.

KABBALAH FINDS US

True love and a successful relationship are the result and the effect of hard spiritual work. An authentic soul mate relationship is not built upon excitement and passion and thrills. Nine times out of ten, the intense excitement and stimulation that usually appears at the beginning of a relationship is just another cocktail, a magic potion laced with poison, handed to us by the Adversary. This passion is what hooks and addicts us. We also call it infatuation.

A rewarding relationship occurs when there is a common spiritual goal, shared spiritual values and a mutual desire to build a relationship

1. upon a spiritual foundation and
2. for the purpose of connecting to the Light of the Creator.

That is the key to any successful relationship. It's never the initial intensity of desire or excitement that makes your heart go pitter patter. As the years go by, those feelings and bodily responses will wane eventually. Only after years of working hard together, and utilizing Resistance to curb your selfishness and work through the ups and downs of the relationship, will true love blossom. Working hard means treating your partner with human dignity and tolerance even when the excitement is missing for the moment. It means remaining dedicated to your partner because there is a larger goal, a bigger picture: the Light of the Creator and the transformation of the world!

Sometimes you may want to strangle her.
Sometimes you may want to hug her.

Sometimes you'll want to kill him.
Sometimes you'll want to kiss him.
Sometimes there will be passion.
Sometimes there will be impatience.
Sometimes there will be excitement.
Sometimes there will be utter boredom.

Working hard means staying the course, rising above these 1 Percent emotions and connecting to the soul level, to the common spiritual goal, even when all your emotions and intellect scream, *What happened? Where did all the passion go?* After you put in these long, hard spiritual years together, then true love, deep fulfillment, and some pretty hot passion emerges . . . and it stays.

Make no mistake: Real, genuine, unconditional love wins out in the end. Think of sports. A sports team doesn't start out the season holding the championship trophy and celebrating victory. Nor do they become champions in the middle of the season. Rather, a team goes through a long, hard-fought season, playing hard in each and every grueling game. The season is then followed by another few "bang-'em-up, knock-'em-down" rounds in the playoffs. Only at the absolute end, when the players can barely stand, can they raise their arms up in victory and be hailed as champions.

The same scenario plays out in a genuine soul mate relationship. All those past lives when you were apart, seeking each other out to no avail, correlate to a season in a sports league. And your present life, in which you finally find each other, is like a playoff round. Only after many seasons of battling and enduring—only after a successful run in the playoffs—can you finally stand up and be declared SOUL MATES!

Whoever is your partner right now may be your path to your true soul mate, or may indeed be your soul mate. If you are without a partner, this is still the most important moment of your life. You are in the game of life right now. You must continue to play and win in order to keep moving forward. You cannot give up. You must keep your eye on the trophy and the final objective at all times. That means finding ways to Resist and transform your desires from selfish acts into acts of sharing and kindness. Not for moral reasons. Do it out of *enlightened greed*. Do it because you want it all!

Utilizing all these kabbalistic tools will give you a rewarding season, no matter what stage of life you find might yourself living in. These tools will hasten the arrival of your soul mate and of great sex. The fact that you are reading this right now means you are pretty close to something substantial. Why? The fact of the matter is we don't find Kabbalah. Kabbalah finds us. We must earn it. We must become worthy in order to discover this knowledge.

Kabbalist Rav Ashlag said very clearly that the wisdom of Kabbalah can safely be revealed in our generation without any fear of wicked, evil, or negative people abusing its power. Why? Because in this day and age, negative souls will actually run away from Kabbalah and its wisdom. Only those whose souls are pure and genuine—despite all the bad habits, sins, and misdeeds that they may have fallen into—will be drawn to this wisdom.

You are here. You are reading these words right now. Therefore, you are close to the ultimate experience of your true soul mate and of sex that rocks the entire cosmos! You can experience great spiritual sex. This life can and will be a winning season.

Just remember, this entire book comes down to this:

> Receiving is our only problem.
> Sharing is our only cure.
> Resistance is our tool to end the problem and receive the cure.

MORE FROM NATIONAL BEST-SELLING AUTHOR YEHUDA BERG

The Power of Kabbalah

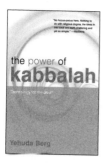

Imagine your life filled with unending joy, purpose, and contentment. Imagine your days infused with pure insight and energy. This is *The Power of Kabbalah*. It is the path from the momentary pleasure that most of us settle for, to the lasting fulfillment that is yours to claim. Your deepest desires are waiting to be realized. But they are not limited to the temporary rush from closing a business deal, the short-term high from drugs, or a passionate sexual relationship that lasts only a few short months.

Wouldn't you like to experience a lasting sense of wholeness and peace that is unshakable, no matter what may be happening around you? Complete fulfillment is the promise of Kabbalah. Within these pages, you will learn how to look at and navigate through life in a whole new way. You will understand your purpose and how to receive the abundant gifts waiting for you. By making a critical transformation from a reactive to a proactive being, you will increase your creative energy, get control of your life, and enjoy new spiritual levels of existence. Kabbalah's ancient teaching is rooted in the perfect union of the physical and spiritual laws already at work in your life. Get ready to experience this exciting realm of awareness, meaning, and joy.

The wonder and wisdom of Kabbalah has influenced the world's leading spiritual, philosophical, religious, and scientific minds. Until today, however, it was hidden away in ancient texts, available only to scholars who knew where to look. Now after many centuries, *The Power of Kabbalah* resides right here in this one remarkable book. Here, at long last is the complete and simple path—actions you can take right now to create the life you desire and deserve.

The 72 Names of God: Technology for the Soul™

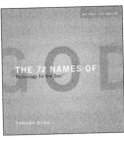

The story of Moses and the Red Sea is well known to almost everyone; it's even been an Academy Award–winning film. What is not known, according to the internationally prominent author Yehuda Berg, is that a state-of-the-art technology is encoded and concealed within that biblical story. This technology is called the 72 Names of God, and it is the key—your key—to ridding yourself of depression, stress, creative stagnation, anger, illness, and other physical and emotional problems. In fact, the 72 Names of God is the oldest, most powerful tool known to mankind—far more powerful than any 21st century high-tech know-how when it comes to eliminating the garbage in your life so that you can wake up and enjoy life each day. Indeed, the 72 Names of God is the ultimate pill for anything and everything that ails you because it strikes at the DNA level of your soul.

The power of the 72 Names of God operates strictly on a soul level, not a physical one. It's about spirituality, not religiosity. Rather than being limited by the differences that divide people, the wisdom of the Names transcends humanity's age-old quarrels and belief systems to deal with the one common bond that unifies all people and nations: the human soul.

It's all here. Everything you wanted to know about the Red String but were afraid to ask!

True Prosperity

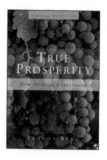

This is a revolution disguised as a book. Based on the secret tools and ancient wisdom of Kabbalah, the world's oldest science of truth, this new volume—by best-selling author Yehuda Berg—harnesses the ultimate truths of the universe as a tool for building prosperity. "Why is it that the people who make the most money out of so called money-making courses are the people who sell the courses?" Berg asks bluntly. "And why do people continue to struggle in anguish in a universe of abundance? And further: "Why do even those who achieve success do so at such bitter cost to their health, happiness, and well-being?" To answer each of these questions, Berg offers a radical overthrow of all our conventional notions of what constitutes money, success, prosperity—and reality! In *True Prosperity*, he launches a total system for achieving prosperity in every aspect of your life. You will learn, step by step, a new operating system for your life—how to become the boss and not the flunky in the business of your life. It is a methodology that you can apply every day and in every minute of your life, beginning now, to unlock the floodgates of money, happiness, fulfilling relationships . . . in a word, everything.

The Red String Book: The Power of Protection

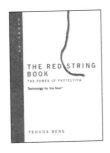

Read the book that everyone is *wearing!*

Discover the ancient technology that empowers and fuels the hugely popular Red String, the most widely recognized tool of kabbalistic wisdom. Yehuda Berg, author of the international best-seller *The 72 Names of God: Technology for the Soul*, continues to reveal the secrets of the world's oldest and most powerful wisdom with his new book, *The Red String Book: The Power of Protection*. Discover the antidote to the negative effects of the dreaded "Evil Eye" in this second book of the Technology for the Soul series.

Find out the real power behind the Red String and why millions of people won't leave home without it.

It's all here. Everything you wanted to know about the Red String but were afraid to ask!

God Does Not Create Miracles. You Do!

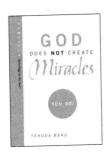

Stop "waiting for a miracle". . . and start making miracles happen!

If you think miracles are one-in-a-million "acts of God," this book will open your eyes and revolutionize your life, starting today! In *God Does Not Create Miracles*, Yehuda Berg gives you the tools to break free of whatever is standing between you and the complete happiness and fulfillment that is your real destiny.

You'll learn why entering the realm of miracles isn't a matter of waiting for a supernatural force to intervene on your behalf. It's about taking action now—using the powerful, practical tools of Kabbalah that Yehuda Berg has brought to the world in his international best sellers *The Power of Kabbalah* and *The 72 Names of God*. Now Yehuda reveals the most astonishing secret of all: the actual formula for creating a connection with the true source of miracles that lies only within yourself.

Discover the Technology for the Soul that really makes miracles happen—and unleash that power to create exactly the life you want and deserve!

The Monster is Real: How to Face Your Fears and Eliminate Them Forever

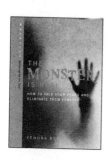

What are you afraid of?

Just admit it! At this very moment, there's something (or maybe lots of things) that you're afraid of. No matter how convincing your fears may seem, this book will show you how to attack and defeat them at their most basic source. In *The Monster Is Real: How to Face Your Fears and Eliminate Them Forever*, Yehuda Berg, author of the international best-seller *The 72 Names of God*, reveals powerful, practical Kabbalistic tools for eliminating fear's inner causes once and for all. If fear in any form is bringing pain into your life, get ready for a hugely positive change. With *The Monster is Real*, another in the Technology for the Soul series, you'll learn how to conquer this age-old problem forever!

FOR TEENS

Life Rules

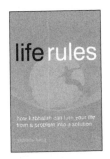

You're a teen. Pretty easy, right? All you've got is social pressure, academic pressure, family pressure, athletic pressure, financial pressure, romantic pressure, and pressure from the thing your biology teacher calls hormones.

And now we want to talk to you about spirituality?

Hang in there. This book isn't one more thing to feel pressured by. In fact, this book is about finding the pressure relief valve that's already built into your soul. And discovering how in the thick of suffering, or what may seem like suffering, you can find never-ending happiness and unlimited joy.

In *LIfe Rules*, Yehuda Berg distills the wisdom of Kabbalah into 13 steps that help you shift from being reactive (that's letting life do it to you) to being proactive (that's you doing it to life).

It's about embracing a spiritual path, but that's different from a religious path. Very different. You won't be shaving your head, giving up parties, or turning in your iPod. What you will be encouraged to do is jump even deeper into life: the fun, the scary, the comfortable, the uncomfortable, all of it. And embrace it.

Your natural state of being is what Kabbalists call *Light-filled*—and through Kabbalistic teachings made easy, personal experiences, and chapter exercises, *Life Rules* will gently challenge you to build the consciousness that will bring you back to this Light. When you do, you will tap into all the mind-blowing abundance and contentment you desire.

NEW FOR KIDS

The 72 Names of God for Kids: A Treasury of Timeless Wisdom

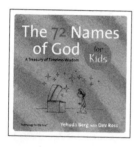

In often seemingly magical ways, the time-less philosophy portrayed in this book will help children overcome their fears and find their way to self-esteem, true friendship, love, and light. The ancient secrets of Kabbalah revealed within these pages will give children a deeper understanding of their innate spiritual selves, along with powerful tools to help them make positive choices throughout their lives. The delightful, original color illustrations were created by the children of Spirituality for Kids who have used these universal lessons to change their own destinies. These are paired with simple and meaning-ful meditations, lessons, stories, poems, and fables inspired by the wisdom of Kabbalah.

MORE PRODUCTS THAT CAN HELP YOU BRING THE WISDOM OF KABBALAH INTO YOUR LIFE

God Wears Lipstick
By Karen Berg

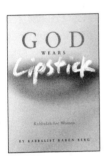

God Wears Lipstick is written exclusively for women (or for men who better want to understand women) by one of the driving forces behind the Kabbalah movement.

For thousands of years, women were banned from studying Kabbalah, the ancient source of wisdom that explains who we are and what our purpose is in this universe.

Karen Berg changed that. She opened the doors of The Kabbalah Centre to anyone who wanted to understand the wisdom of Kabbalah and brought Light to these people.

In *God Wears Lipstick*, Karen Berg shares that wisdom with us, especially as it affects you and your relationships. She reveals a woman's special place in the universe and why women have a spiritual advantage over men. She explains how to find your soulmate and your purpose in life. She empowers you to become a better human being as you connect to the Light, and she then gives you the tools for living and loving.

Becoming Like God
By Michael Berg

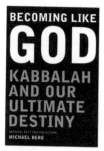

At the age of 16, kabbalistic scholar Michael Berg began the herculean task of translating *The Zohar*, Kabbalah's chief text, from its original Aramaic into its first complete English translation. *The Zohar*, which consists of 23 volumes, is considered a compendium of virtually all information pertaining to the universe, and its wisdom is only beginning to be verified today.

During the ten years he worked on *The Zohar*, Michael Berg discovered the long-lost secret for which humanity has searched for more than 5,000 years: how to achieve our ultimate destiny. *Becoming Like God* reveals the transformative method by which people can actually break free of what is called "ego nature" to achieve total joy and lasting life.

Berg puts forth the revolutionary idea that for the first time in history, an opportunity is being made available to humankind: an opportunity to Become Like God.

The Secret
By Michael Berg

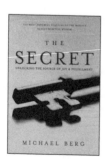

Like a jewel that has been painstakingly cut and polished, *The Secret* reveals life's essence in its most concise and powerful form. Michael Berg begins by showing you how our everyday understanding of our purpose in the world is literally backwards. Whenever there is pain in our lives—indeed, whenever there is anything less than complete joy and fulfillment—this basic misunderstanding is the reason.

The Essential Zohar
By Rav Berg

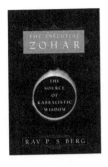

The Zohar has traditionally been known as the world's most esoteric and profound spiritual document, but Kabbalist Rav Berg, this generation's greatest living Kabbalist, has dedicated his life to making this wisdom universally available. The vast wisdom and Light of *The Zohar* came into being as a gift to all humanity, and *The Essential Zohar* at last explains this gift to the world.

The Power of You
By Rav Berg

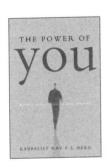

For the past 5,000 years, neither science nor psychology has been able to solve the fundamental problem of chaos in people's lives.

Now, one man is providing the answer. He is Kabbalist Rav Berg.

Beneath the pain and chaos that disrupts our lives, Kabbalist Rav Berg brings to light a hidden realm of order, purpose, and unity. Revealed is a universe in which mind becomes master over matter—a world in which God, human thought, and the entire cosmos are mysteriously interconnected.

Join this generation's premier kabbalist on a mind-bending journey along the cutting edge of reality. Peer into the vast reservoir of spiritual wisdom that is Kabbalah, where the secrets of creation, life, and death have remained hidden for thousands of years.

Wheels of a Soul
By Rav Berg

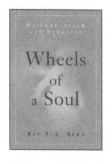

In *Wheels of a Soul*, Kabbalist Rav Berg reveals the keys to answering these and many more questions that lie at the heart of our existence as human beings. Specifically, Rav Berg explains why we must acknowledge and explore the lives we have already lived in order to understand the life we are living today . . .

Make no mistake: *you have been here before*. Reincarnation is a fact—and just as science is now beginning to recognize that time and space may be nothing but illusions, Rav Berg shows why death itself is the greatest illusion of all.

In this book you learn much more than the answers to these questions. You will understand your true purpose in the world and discover tools to identify your life's soul mate. Read *Wheels of a Soul* and let one of the greatest kabbalistic masters of our time change your life forever.

THE ZOHAR

"Bringing *The Zohar* from near oblivion to wide accessibility has taken many decades. It is an achievement of which we are truly proud and grateful."

—Michael Berg

Composed more than 2,000 years ago, *The Zohar* is a set of 23 books, a commentary on biblical and spiritual matters in the form of conversations among spiritual masters. But to describe *The Zohar* only in physical terms is greatly misleading. In truth, *The Zohar* is nothing less than a powerful tool for achieving the most important purposes of our lives. It was given to all humankind by the Creator to bring us protection, to connect us with the Creator's Light, and ultimately to fulfill our birthright of true spiritual transformation.

More than eighty years ago, when The Kabbalah Centre was founded, *The Zohar* had virtually disappeared from the world. Few people in the general population had ever heard of it. Whoever sought to read it—in any country, in any language, at any price—faced a long and futile search.

Today all this has changed. Through the work of The Kabbalah Centre and the editorial efforts of Michael Berg, *The Zohar* is now being brought to the world, not only in the original Aramaic language but also in English.

The new English *Zohar* provides everything for connecting to this sacred text on all levels: the original Aramaic text for scanning; an English translation; and clear, concise commentary for study and learning.

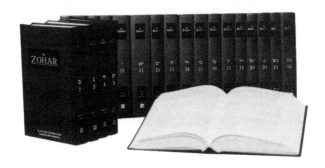

THE KABBALAH CENTRE

The International Leader in the Education of Kabbalah

Since its founding, The Kabbalah Centre has had a single mission: to improve and transform people's lives by bringing the power and wisdom of Kabbalah to all who wish to partake of it.

Through the lifelong efforts of Kabbalists Rav and Karen Berg, and the great spiritual lineage of which they are a part, an astonishing 3.5 million people around the world have already been touched by the powerful teachings of Kabbalah. And each year, the numbers are growing!

• • • •

If you were inspired by this book in any way and would like to know how you can continue to enrich your life through the wisdom of Kabbalah, here is what you can do next:

Call 1-800-KABBALAH where trained instructors are available 18 hours a day. These dedicated people are willing to answer any and all questions about Kabbalah and help guide you along in your effort to learn more.

May the words in this book speak to your soul
and enlighten your life.

May you find true love with your soul mate.

Jim and Shelley Haim-Sarvey